WORKING SAFELY IN HEALTH CARE

A Quick Reference

DEBORAH L. FELL-CARLSON,

RN, MSPH, COHN-S, HEM

THOMSON

DELMAR LEARNING

Australia • Brazil • Canada • Mexico • Singapore • Spain • United Kingdom • United States

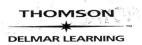

THOMSON

DELMAR LEARNING

Working Safely in Health Care: A Quick Reference
by Deborah Fell-Carlson

Vice President, Health Care Business Unit:
William Brottmiller

Director of Learning Solutions:
Matthew Kane

Managing Editor:
Marah Bellegarde

Acquisitions Editor:
Matthew Seeley

Product Manager:
Jadin Babin-Kavanaugh

Editorial Assistant:
Megan Tarquinio

Marketing Director:
Jennifer McAvey

Marketing Manager:
Michele McTighe

Marketing Coordinator:
Andrea Eobstel

Production Director:
Carolyn Miller

Content Project Manager:
Anne Sherman

Art Director:
Jack Pendleton

Notice to the Reader

CONTENTS

CHAPTER 5

PART 2

CHAPTER 6

CHAPTER 7

PART 3

CHAPTER 8

CHAPTER 9

CHAPTER 10

CHAPTER 17

CHAPTER 18

CHAPTER 19

INTRODUCTION

This Quick Reference version of *Working Safely in Health Care: A Practical Guide* is designed to provide vital health and workplace safety information at the fingertips of health care workers in all settings. We have taken the key concepts from the main textbook and bound them into this smaller, more portable volume for your convenience.

Essential figures and tables have been retained with the original figure and table numbers to allow you to easily refer to the main text if additional information is needed. Chapter features, Web links, reference lists, and in-depth explanations of concepts found in the main text have been omitted in this Quick Reference. This tool is created for the busy caregiver who has a good grasp of the concepts presented in the main text, but needs a quick and easy way to access key safety information while on the job.

The focus of the main textbook and this Quick Reference is not regulatory compliance, but on best practices, sound prevention principles, and interventions that do not change with the next round of regulatory rule-making. This Quick Reference is not intended to supplant facility policy. Safe work practices and regulatory compliance related to client and caregiver safety remain an individual and organizational responsibility. It is always a good idea to consult facility legal counsel with policy-related questions related to safety and health.

Some interventions presented in the main textbook and this Quick Reference may include new ways to deliver care, such as the use of lift equipment to move and transfer clients. Equipment and devices depicted in images throughout these publications are provided for illustrative purposes only, and their depiction should not be construed as an approval or endorsement, or a representation of the efficacy or safety, of a particular product or device.

The author and the publisher hope that this Quick Reference version of *Working Safely in Health Care: A Practical Guide* will provide answers to questions that may arise on the job, and assist you in providing a higher level of care, for your patients as well as for yourself and the health care team.

SECTION I

LAYING THE FOUNDATION

CHAPTER

1

CARING FOR THE CAREGIVER— A FRESH APPROACH TO HEALTH CARE SAFETY

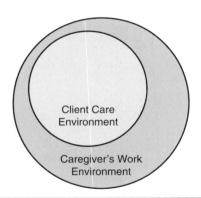

FIGURE 1-4 An integrated approach to health care safety. *Because the client care environment and the caregiver work environment overlap, safety improvements in the caregiver's work environment can have a positive impact on client safety, as well.*

A SYSTEMS APPROACH TO SAFETY IN HEALTH CARE

A **safety system** can be thought of as an approach that attempts to address the safety impact of interrelating factors within the workplace rather than focusing only on hazards. These safety factors include **social aspects** (how individuals and departments interact and relate with each other) and **technical aspects** (how individuals interact and relate with their work environment and the hazards present within that environment).

Social Aspects of Safety

Trust, respect, and communication can be viewed as social aspects of safety. Caregivers who have a trusting and respectful relationship are more likely to report a minor incident or **near-miss,** perhaps preventing a serious mishap. Near-misses are incidents with the potential for injury or property damage that were averted. Open, candid communication enriches the safety system, as freedom to speak up without fear of being ridiculed or disciplined has been shown to improve client safety and quality of care.

Technical Aspects of Safety

Safety systems have an equally important technical aspect, summarized in the following paragraphs. A system of policies, procedures, or activities designed to address the technical aspects of a safety issue is commonly called a **safety program.** Safety programs can be ongoing or may have a predetermined end point.

Work-Site Hazard Analysis, Hazard Prevention, and Control

Work-site hazard analysis is the process of identifying and analyzing existing hazards to determine their severity. Once the hazard has been identified and analyzed, measures are taken to control or eliminate it.

Safety and Health Training

Training blends social and technical aspects of safety and health. Minimal training requirements are established by certain government agencies, but employers may provide additional training based on hazards unique to the work environment.

Incident Analysis

Incident analysis (sometimes called accident analysis) is a systematic process that seeks to discover the underlying factors contributing to the incident so they can be addressed to prevent recurrence. The first priority in the event of any injury is the care and continued safety of the injured, but the incident analysis begins as soon as possible after care has been provided, because as time passes, important details can be lost.

Embracing Change

Change is difficult, especially in health care. It is estimated to take an average of 17 years for new clinical evidence to be effectively transferred into practice, a process called **knowledge transfer.** Without management commitment and caregiver involvement to hasten the process, this delay can become a barrier to rapid improvements in health care safety.

OSHA AND HEALTH CARE SAFETY

The mission of the **Occupational Safety and Health Administration (OSHA)** is to protect the safety and health of America's workers through regulations, training, and partnerships. OSHA often uses research findings provided by the **National Institute for Occupational Safety and Health (NIOSH)** to set standards for workplace safety and health. NIOSH is an agency within the Centers for Disease Control and Prevention (CDC) with a mission to conduct research, education, and training to assist OSHA and employers.

OSHA Standards and the General Duty Clause

The intent of the Occupational Safety and Health Act of 1970 was to provide workplaces "free of recognized hazards." The Act covers all U.S. businesses engaged in commerce, with few exceptions. The original Act did not directly cover government workplaces at any level. By executive order, coverage was extended to federal workers in 1980. In addition, many states regulate government workplaces at the state level through state OSHA rules, which must be at least as stringent as the federal rules.

Congress penned a provision in the Act to cover "all recognized hazards." This section of the Act is often called the "General Duty Clause," and it outlines the general duties of the employer and employee in maintaining a safe and healthful workplace.

See Tables 17-2 and 17-3 in this guide for employee rights and responsibilities under OSHA.

Duties under the General Duty Clause of the Occupational Safety and Health Act of 1970

(a) *Each employer—*
   (1) *shall furnish to each of his employees employment and a place of employment which are free from recognized hazards that are causing or are likely to cause death or serious physical harm to his employees;*
   (2) *shall comply with occupational safety and health standards promulgated under this Act.*
(b) *Each employee shall comply with occupational safety and health standards and all rules, regulations, and orders issued pursuant to this Act which are applicable to his own actions and conduct.*

The Joint Commission Environment of Care Standards

The Joint Commission **environment of care (EOC)** standards provide a framework for a comprehensive organization-wide program to improve safety for workers, clients, visitors, students, and others who share the environment.

The Joint Commission separates the EOC into seven broad categories, depicted in Table 1-1 along with examples of caregiver responsibilities for each.

TABLE 1-1   The Seven Environment of Care Areas and Examples of Caregiver Activities

Environment of Care Category	Program Goal	Examples of Related Caregiver Activities
Safety	Minimize risk of injury to clients, visitors, and staff.	• Observe work environment and report hazards or safety concerns promptly. • Participate on organization's safety committee. • Attend safety training. • Use safe work practices, including appropriate lifts and client-handling devices. • Report all injuries promptly. • Know policies and procedures.
Security management	Physical and personal safety of staff; protection of material and property is secondary.	• Wear identification badge. • Report hostile or suspicious activity. • Participate in infant-abduction drills. • Exit with a coworker when leaving after dark. • Secure personal valuables and sensitive equipment during the shift. • Secure medications, needles, and syringes. • Know bomb-threat procedures. • Participate in workplace violence prevention training and other security training. • Know policies and procedures.
Emergency management	Management of situations that disrupt care. Includes contingencies for natural and human-made disasters. Phases: preparedness, **mitigation** (activities to minimize or reduce loss in the event of a disaster or catastrophe), response, and recovery (returning to normal operations).	• Be familiar with the evacuation plan and your role in the overall emergency management plan in your organization. • Become familiar with characteristics of hazards most likely to occur in your region. • Seek knowledge on actions necessary to protect your home and your family and make appropriate plans in the event you are separated from them.

(continued)

TABLE 1-1 (continued)

Environment of Care Category	Program Goal	Examples of Related Caregiver Activities
		• Participate in disaster drills and other emergency management training.
		• Know policies and procedures.
Hazardous materials and waste management	Safe storage, handling, and disposal of chemical, radiological, and biological materials and wastes.	• Know the location and understand content of the Material Safety Data Sheets (MSDSs) for chemicals used in workplace.
		• Use proper protective equipment as prescribed on MSDS.
		• Ensure that labeling is present on all containers.
		• Use proper disposal methods.
		• Empty sharps containers when three-fourths full.
		• Attend hazard communication training and other safety training on substances used in the workplace.
		• Know policies and procedures.
Utilities	Supply adequate air quality, lighting, water, and power to the environment.	• Know location of utility shutoffs, including oxygen shutoffs.
		• Know which outlets and equipment systems have generator backup in the event of power failure.
		• Unplug equipment when not in use.
		• Know reporting procedures.
		• Know policies and procedures.
Fire safety	Provide a fire-safe environment.	• Keep hallways free of clutter and equipment.
		• Do not block exit doorways.
		• Know fire policies and procedures, including location of nearest fire pull and fire extinguisher.
		• Know primary and alternative exit routes.
		• Know where clients are to be taken in the event of a fire.
		• Know assembly areas and how clients and staff are to be accounted for.
Medical equipment	Training, use, storage, and care of medical equipment to ensure that it does not endanger clients or staff.	• Maintain proficiency on all equipment.
		• If a problem is found, take equipment out of service and tag it.
		• Report equipment problems promptly.
		• If qualified to make a repair or conduct equipment inspection, lock out equipment beforehand to prevent unexpected startup.
		• Know policies and procedures.

Adapted from *The Environment of Care Handbook.* Oakbrook Terrace, IL: Joint Commission, 1998; *Protecting Those Who Serve: Health Care Worker Safety.* Oakbrook Terrace, IL: Joint Commission Resources, 2005.

CHAPTER

2

UNDERSTANDING HAZARDS AND CONTROLS IN HEALTH CARE

INTRODUCTION

Caregivers work in environments where there are many hazards that can result in injuries and illnesses. Safety measures that are used to decrease the risk of injury in health care environments not only decrease risk for caregivers, but also decrease risk for clients. Caregivers can take charge of their own safety and can make sure they are aware of and know how to control the hazards in their workplace.

HAZARD SEVERITY AND RISK

Exposure to a hazard does not always end in an adverse outcome or mishap; rather it is the opportunity to receive a hazard **dose.** Risk of injury or illness can be influenced by the actual dose received, the severity of the hazard, and the unique characteristics of individuals (see Table 2-1). The concept of potential dose is a way of measuring exposure to a hazard. Potential dose considers the duration of the exposure to the hazard (how long), the frequency of the exposure to the hazard (how often), and the amount of the hazard involved in the exposure (how much).

The severity of the hazard is the capacity of the hazard to cause a serious injury, illness, or death. Simply put, just how bad is the hazard? Some

TABLE 2-1   Factors Affecting Risk of Injury

Dose	The amount of chemical or other substance actually received by the body as a result of an exposure	Potential dose in exposure evaluation considers: How often (frequency)? How long (duration)? How much (amount)?
Severity, or, in the case of chemicals, the toxicity	The capacity of the hazard to cause a serious injury or illness	Considers: How bad could it be?
Individual differences	Health effects related to unique individual characteristics	Considers: allergies, medications, gender, body size, general health, lifestyle habits, etc.

chemicals are more toxic than others and present a more severe hazard in the event of exposure.

Finally, the uniqueness of individuals may also affect risk. Whether or not a caregiver or client is prone to allergies, is taking medications, is male or female, or is large or small can impact risk. General health and lifestyle habits also impact risk.

CONTROLS

Hazard controls are methods used to prevent a hazard from doing as much harm as it could. Control strategies are based on the specific hazard and the conditions in the work environment.

INJURIES AND NEAR-MISS INCIDENTS

Near-miss incidents are events that occur without injury. Attention to events that did not result in a mishap, but could have, can prevent future incidents. Many facilities keep track of injuries and near-misses and analyze them to determine their cause.

IDENTIFYING HAZARDS, ASSESSING RISK, AND DETERMINING CONTROLS

Many hazards in the health care workplace are obvious, such as a cord in the walkway. However, some hazards are not as easy to recognize. Some chemicals can give off vapors that cause illness, either immediately or over time. Certain substances, such as latex, can cause an irritant or allergic reaction in some workers but not in others. Each is an example of a type of hazard that might be difficult to recognize and even more difficult to evaluate and control.

TABLE 2-2   Job Safety Analysis (JSA)

1. Break down each job task into steps.
2. Identify hazards associated with each step.
3. Determine actions necessary to eliminate or minimize hazards.

Job Safety Analysis

Job safety analysis (JSA), sometimes called "job hazard analysis," is a method of hazard identification and control that is easy to learn and is appropriate for many caregiver activities. The process is summarized in Table 2-2. See Table 2-3 for an example.

Learning about the appropriate control measures may take some effort and may require collaboration with, and research by, supervisors, safety professionals, and other caregivers.

TABLE 2-3   Sample Job Safety Analysis (JSA) Worksheet

High-Risk Job: Registered Nurse, Certified Nursing Assistant

High-Risk Job Task Elements	Hazards Associated with Task Elements	Solutions to Control Job Hazards
High-Risk Task: Pulling Totally Dependent Client Up in Bed		
Element 1: Roll client to left side (Caregiver 1 and 2)	Lifting/pushing up on heavy load, reaching, bending, awkward posture	Make sure bed is at proper working height with side rail down
Element 2: Insert draw sheet under client (Caregiver 1)	Lifting/supporting heavy load, awkward posture, reaching, bending	Make sure bed is at proper working height with side rail down
Element 3: Roll client to right side (Caregiver 1 and 2)	Lifting/pushing/pulling heavy load, reaching, bending, awkward posture	Make sure bed is at proper working height with side rail down
Element 4: Pull draw sheet out on other side (Caregiver 2)	Lifting/supporting heavy load, reaching, bending, awkward posture, pulling	Make sure bed is at proper working height with side rail down
Element 5: Roll draw sheet in hands (Caregiver 1 and 2)		Make sure bed is at proper working height with side rail down
Element 6: Grasp draw sheet (Caregiver 1 and 2)	Stress on fingers and hands from pinched grip	Make sure bed is at proper working height with side rail down
		Grasp draw sheet with entire hand

(continued)

TABLE 2-3 (continued)		
Element 7: Pull client up in bed with draw sheet (Caregiver 1 and 2)	Lifting/pulling heavy load, reaching, awkward posture	Use friction-reducing device (slide board, roller board, slip sheets, etc.) or mechanical lifting equipment with repositioning sling instead of draw sheet to decrease load and stress on caregivers. Make sure bed is at proper working height with side rail down.
Element 8: Roll client to right side (Caregiver 2)	Lifting/pushing heavy load, reaching, bending, awkward posture	Make sure bed is at proper working height with side rail down
Element 9 . . . (Continue removal process)		

Controlling Hazards in Health Care Environments—The Hierarchy of Controls

The **hierarchy of controls** ranks hazard controls by the method and degree of protection they provide. This classification system aids safety professionals in selecting the most appropriate and effective control or combination of controls for each specific hazard in the work environment. (see Table 2-4).

Hazard Elimination

Hazard elimination is the most effective way to reduce risk in any workplace. Hazard elimination includes the substitution of an alternative for the hazard or the total removal of the hazard from the work environment. Although hazard elimination is certainly the best way to reduce risk, it is sometimes not feasible.

Engineering Controls

If a hazard cannot be removed or a substitution found, then **engineering controls** are the next best control method to reduce risk. These controls lessen exposure by either reducing the hazard at its source or isolating the worker from the hazard. Engineering controls modify the work environment. Engineering controls do not eliminate the task completely, but they do reduce the risk substantially.

Administrative Controls and Work-Practice Controls

An **administrative control** is a method of controlling hazards by using policies, procedures, training, supervision, and communication to reduce risk factors associated with the hazard by prescribing safe work practices,

TABLE 2-4   Hierarchy of Controls

Control Strategy	Description	Example
Hazard elimination	Involves the substitution of an alternative for the hazard or the total removal of the hazard from the work environment. Most effective way to reduce risk.	Scale integrated into the bed eliminates high-risk transfer task to weigh client. A needleless intravenous system substituted for a hazardous sharp.
Engineering controls	Reduce risk by modifying the work environment or device being used. Lessen exposure by reducing the hazard at its source or isolating the individual from the hazard. Next best control method after hazard elimination.	Mechanical lifting equipment modifies the work environment; use of the lift transfers the weight of the client to the lift. A retractable needle modifies the device and removes the source of a potential puncture wound. An exhaust fan automatically turns on when the light is turned on.
Administrative controls	Change the way an activity is performed in order to reduce risk. Includes use of hygiene practices, housekeeping, maintenance, or changes in procedures or processes to control hazards.	Good hand-washing practices decrease risk of infection (work-practice control). In a long-term care facility, scheduling clients for therapy at different times during the morning staggers the high-risk transfer tasks throughout the morning (administrative control).
Personal protective equipment (PPE)	Barriers worn by workers to reduce the possibility of exposure to a hazard. Used when other control methods do not sufficiently control the hazard, in combination with other controls, when engineering controls are in the process of being introduced, and in emergency situations.	Respirators protect caregivers from exposure to airborne infectious disease. Gloves protect from bloodborne pathogens. Protective clothing during surgical procedures protects caregivers from exposure to blood and protects clients from infectious disease that may be carried by the caregiver.

also called work-practice controls. The hazard is still present, and can cause harm if the controls are not followed.

Personal Protective Equipment

Personal protective equipment (PPE) typically includes items of clothing that serve as a barrier between the caregiver and the hazard. Examples include respirators, gloves, safety goggles and glasses, splash guards, helmets, safety shoes, earplugs, and aprons. PPE may be used as a last resort, when engineering and administrative controls do not adequately control a hazard, or in combination with other controls to provide additional protection. PPE can also be used when engineering controls are in the process of being introduced, and in emergency situations. The safety professional should be consulted to ensure that using PPE is the appropriate control for a hazard and that the appropriate PPE has been selected. Since caregivers have unique physical characteristics, PPE must be individually and properly fitted.

COMMON HEALTH CARE HAZARDS

In order to better understand workplace hazards, they are grouped into categories (see Table 2-5). It is important to note that combinations of these can be found in the workplace.

TABLE 2-5 Examples of Common Health Care Hazards

Categories	Description	Examples
Environmental hazards	Unsafe conditions in the workplace	Slip, trip, fall hazards; uneven work surfaces; poor room design; clutter; cramped working space; inefficient equipment; lack of storage; inadequate equipment maintenance
Physical hazards	Agents that can cause physical injury and tissue trauma	Temperature (heat and cold), radiation, noise, explosive objects or substances
Chemical hazards	May have toxic effects through inhalation, absorption through the skin, or ingestion. Some irritate the skin on contact.	Formaldehyde, chemotherapeutic agents, alcohol, disinfectants, floor-care products
Biological/infectious hazards	May cause infection through inhalation, direct contact with skin or mucosa, skin puncture, or through ingestion (eating or drinking)	Bacteria, viruses, fungi, and other living microorganisms. Pulmonary tuberculosis, *Staphylococcus aureus*, and mold are examples.
Ergonomic (musculoskeletal) hazards	Unsafe workplace design and lack of appropriate client- and material-handling tools and equipment contributing to	Activities that require lifting heavy loads, twisting, bending, reaching, holding body parts and other materials for long periods,

(continued)

TABLE 2-5   (continued)

Categories	Description	Examples
	increased risk of musculoskeletal disorders. Poor lighting, excessive vibration, and noise are also considered ergonomic hazards.	standing for long periods, pushing, pulling, awkward postures, repetitive motions. High-detail work in dimly lighted area, noisy environment.
Psychosocial hazards	Stressors in the workplace causing workplace anxiety and emotional fatigue	Providing constant emotional support, coping with emergency situations, workplace violence, verbal and physical assaults, inadequate staffing, lack of supervisor support, shift work

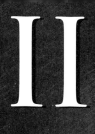

SECTION II

HAZARDS AND CONTROLS IN HEALTH CARE

PART 1

PREVENTING MUSCULOSKELETAL INJURIES IN HEALTH CARE

CHAPTER

3

PERFORMING CLINICAL SUPPORT TASKS SAFELY

WHAT ARE MUSCULOSKELETAL DISORDERS?

A **musculoskeletal disorder** is a condition that involves the muscles, tendons, ligaments, nerves, blood vessels, spinal discs, or joints of the hands and wrists, arms, neck, shoulder, back, and legs.

Musculoskeletal disorders can range from **acute** to **chronic** disabling conditions. An acute injury or condition may be mild to severe, but is typically of short duration.

Chronic injuries or conditions are of long duration and may cause a lasting change in the body. Examples include **muscle strains** and **ligament sprains, tendonitis, tenosynovitis, low-back pain, tension neck syndrome, bursitis, carpal tunnel syndrome,** and **degenerative arthritis.** See Table 3-1 for definitions of these conditions. Symptoms of musculoskeletal disorders may include persistent pain or discomfort, soft-tissue swelling, stiffness, numbness and tingling of the affected body part, or restriction of joint movement.

Musculoskeletal disorders may also result from the accumulation of tissue damage from many small injuries, or **microtraumas,** or from overuse of a body part over weeks, months, or years. These are called **cumulative musculoskeletal disorders.** Refer to Table 3-2 for other common terms for cumulative musculoskeletal disorders.

TABLE 3-1   Examples of Types of Musculoskeletal Disorders and Definitions

Muscle strain	Damage to muscle fibers from repeated use or prolonged static posture without sufficient rest (e.g., low-back pain)
Ligament sprain	Damage to ligament fibers from moving or twisting a joint beyond its normal range
Tendonitis	Inflammation of a tendon (e.g., shoulder tendonitis and rotator cuff injuries, epicondylitis or tennis elbow, de Quervain's disease)
Tenosynovitis	Inflammation of a tendon and its sheath (e.g., in the wrists, hands, or fingers)
Tension neck syndrome	Irritation of the muscles and tendons where the last neck vertebra meets the first midback vertebra
Bursitis	Irritation and inflammation of bursa in the shoulders
Carpal tunnel syndrome	Swelling and entrapment of the median nerve in the wrist
Degenerative arthritis	Wearing out of joints, vertebrae, discs, facets, or other structures over time. Also called "osteoarthritis."

Work-related musculoskeletal disorders (WRMSDs) are musculoskeletal disorders such as the disorders listed in Table 3-1 that may be caused or aggravated by excessive exposure to certain risk factors that occur when performing tasks at work. WRMSDs can cause severe, long-term symptoms if not treated promptly and correctly.

Whether caused by tasks performed at work or off the job, musculoskeletal disorders can make normal work routines uncomfortable and even painful. This can lead to stress or dissatisfaction at work, reduced productivity, the inability to perform some or all job tasks, and even difficulty with activities at home.

UNDERSTANDING RISK FACTORS FOR WRMSDs

Risk factors include physical factors that contribute to cumulative WRMSDs. The primary risk factors for musculoskeletal disorders are awkward postures, static postures, forceful exertions, and repetition. One or several of these risk factors may be present in a single job task or multiple job tasks.

Exposure to other risk factors such as **contact stress** and **vibration** may contribute to musculoskeletal disorders. **Environmental factors** such as hot or cold temperatures or poor lighting and glare may also be contributing factors.

TABLE 3-2   Other Commonly Used Terms for Cumulative Musculoskeletal Disorders

Cumulative trauma disorders

Repetitive trauma disorders

Repetitive strain injuries

Repetitive motion disorders

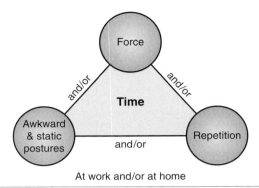

FIGURE 3-1 Primary risk factors for musculoskeletal disorders. *(Concept developed by Lynda Enos. Courtesy of the Oregon Nurses Association, Bay Area Hospital, University of Oregon Labor Education and Research Center, and Oregon OSHA)*

The level of risk for injury depends on the severity or magnitude of the risk factor(s) present in a job task, the frequency of the activity or how often you are exposed to one or more of the risk factors, and for how long—the duration—you are exposed when performing job tasks. Figure 3-1 illustrates the relationship between the primary risk factors and the duration of exposure.

Job tasks, working conditions, or non-work activities that combine risk factors will increase the risk for musculoskeletal disorders. When the musculoskeletal system is exposed to a combination of these risk factors without sufficient recovery or rest time, damage occurs. This wear and tear process eventually causes physical symptoms such as pain and swelling. Figure 3-2 illustrates this concept. Examples of awkward postures, forceful exertions, and contact stress are illustrated in Figures 3-3 through 3-5.

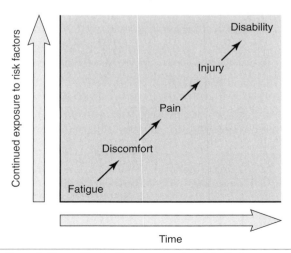

FIGURE 3-2 Cumulative effect of exposure to risk factors over time. *(Concept developed by Lynda Enos. Courtesy of the Oregon Nurses Association, Bay Area Hospital, University of Oregon Labor Education and Research Center, and Oregon OSHA)*

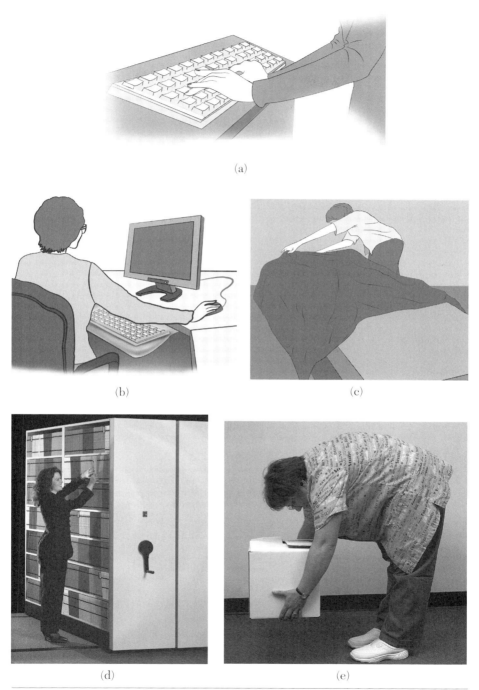

FIGURE 3-3 Examples of awkward postures: (a) wrist extension; (b) extended reach away from the body; (c) extreme forward bending and twisting of the back, extended reach; (d) reaching over shoulder height; (e) extreme bending.

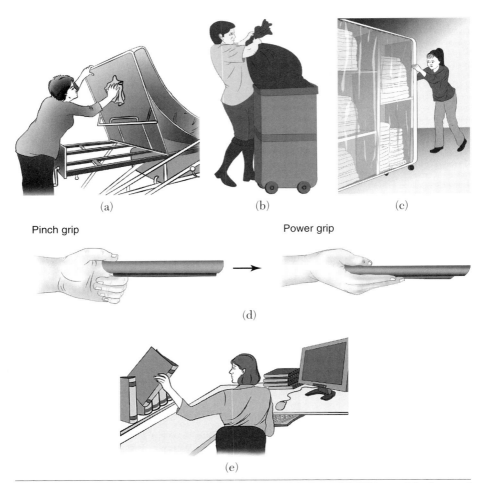

Pinch grip

Power grip

(a) (b) (c)

(d)

(e)

FIGURE 3-4 Examples of forceful exertions: (a) forceful lifting with forward bending; (b) forceful lifting, high grip force, and awkward posture of the back and arms; (c) forceful exertion when pushing with high grip force and awkward posture of the arms; (d) examples of pinch grip and power grip; (e) forceful grip and awkward postures of the arm and neck.

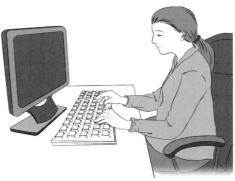

FIGURE 3-5 Contact stress on the wrists and arms from the edge of a desk.

Duration of Exposure to Risk Factors for WRMSDs

The risk of injury may be increased by a long duration of exposure to the task and by the intensity and combination of risk factors. Taking breaks, limiting overtime, and varying tasks to use different muscle groups can help reduce the duration of exposure to risk factors. If exposure continues over weeks, months, and years with insufficient recovery time, the severity of the WRMSD may increase.

PREVENTING AND REDUCING RISK FACTORS FOR WRMSDS

The risk factors in job tasks described in the previous section of this chapter occur because of a poor match between the job task and the users' or caregivers' physical capabilities and body dimensions.

Ergonomics

Ergonomics involves fitting the physical and cognitive demands of the job to the caregiver to prevent human error and injuries such as WRMSDs and to improve caregiver and client comfort. (See Figure 3-6.)

Ergonomics Controls

Risk factors contributing to WRMSDs can be reduced or controlled by using the hierarchy of controls. The most effective approach to controlling musculoskeletal risk factors is to use engineering controls. Engineering controls involve eliminating or minimizing exposure to risk factors by redesigning, changing, or modifying the physical properties of the task, tools, equipment, or work area layout.

Ergonomics is

"Fitting the Job to the Worker"

not

"Fitting the Worker to the Job"

The goal of ergonomics is to design equipment, job tasks, and work environments so that a majority of employees can perform tasks safely and comfortably

---

FIGURE 3-6 Defining "ergonomics."

```
Engineering Controls
+
Safe Work Practices
+
Administrative
Controls
=
Reduce the Risk of Injury for
Caregivers and Clients
```

FIGURE 3-7 Ergonomics controls. *(Courtesy of Lynda Enos and the Oregon Nurses Association, Bay Area Hospital, University of Oregon Labor Education and Research Center, and Oregon OSHA)*

If risk factors cannot be eliminated or minimized by using engineering controls, caregiver exposure to risk factors should be reduced using administrative and work-practice controls. These controls use policies, procedures, training, supervision, communication, and safe work practices to reduce the amount of time (duration), the frequency of the activity (how often), or the severity or magnitude of the risk factor(s) that a caregiver is exposed to when performing a job task. See Figure 3-7.

There are only a few examples of personal protective equipment (PPE) that effectively provide a barrier between the caregiver and a WRMSD risk factor. Knee pads and antivibration gloves are examples.

Some facilities provide back belts to caregivers in an attempt to help prevent injuries. The National Institute for Occupational Safety and Health (NIOSH) has published materials to caution employers and employees about the lack of evidence supporting the use of back belts as an injury control measure for lifting tasks.

APPLYING ERGONOMICS TO THE HEALTH CARE WORK ENVIRONMENT

Refer to Table 3-3 for a list of core principles that can be used to reduce risk factors for WRMSDs.

Maintain Neutral Posture

Neutral postures (postures, typically near the midrange of joint range of motion, that are the body's strongest and most balanced positions for performing job tasks) reduce physical stress on musculoskeletal structures and optimize blood flow to the musculoskeletal system. Figure 3-8 describes how to achieve neutral postures in a standing position.

TABLE 3-3   Applying Ergonomics to Your Work Environment: Core Principles

1. Use neutral postures when performing job tasks
2. Reduce static postures
3. Reduce forces and loads
4. Minimize contact stress
5. Reduce repetitions
6. Maintain a comfortable environment
7. Use safe work practices

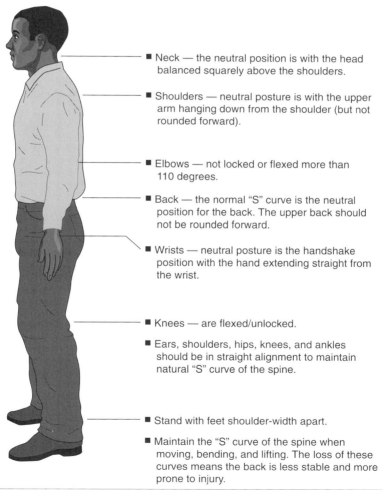

- Neck — the neutral position is with the head balanced squarely above the shoulders.

- Shoulders — neutral posture is with the upper arm hanging down from the shoulder (but not rounded forward).

- Elbows — not locked or flexed more than 110 degrees.

- Back — the normal "S" curve is the neutral position for the back. The upper back should not be rounded forward.

- Wrists — neutral posture is the handshake position with the hand extending straight from the wrist.

- Knees — are flexed/unlocked.

- Ears, shoulders, hips, knees, and ankles should be in straight alignment to maintain natural "S" curve of the spine.

- Stand with feet shoulder-width apart.

- Maintain the "S" curve of the spine when moving, bending, and lifting. The loss of these curves means the back is less stable and more prone to injury.

FIGURE 3-8   Neutral posture for work performed in a standing position. *(Concept courtesy of Lynda Enos)*

The caregiver **workstation** is an area or work space where a particular task is performed. To maintain a safe work environment, the caregiver must make continual adjustments to maintain neutral posture as different tasks are performed in a variety of workstations.

Adjust Work Height

Work performed at the proper height, within easy reach, and in line of sight facilitates neutral postures. As a general guideline, most tasks performed at a workstation, such as using the computer or working at the bedside, should be performed at elbow height. Writing tasks may be performed at about 2 inches above elbow height. Tasks that require force to be applied in a downward direction are best performed on a work surface below elbow height. Figure 3-9 shows working heights for specific tasks.

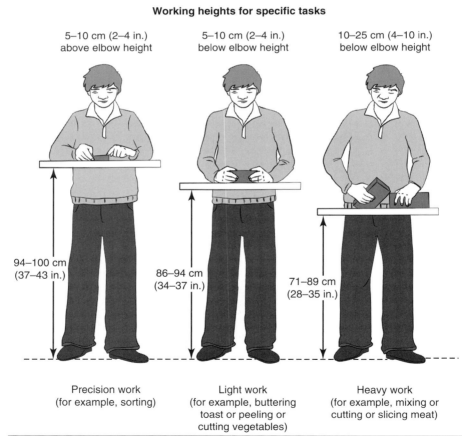

Working heights for specific tasks

5–10 cm (2–4 in.) above elbow height	5–10 cm (2–4 in.) below elbow height	10–25 cm (4–10 in.) below elbow height

94–100 cm (37–43 in.)

86–94 cm (34–37 in.)

71–89 cm (28–35 in.)

Precision work (for example, sorting)

Light work (for example, buttering toast or peeling or cutting vegetables)

Heavy work (for example, mixing or cutting or slicing meat)

FIGURE 3-9 Examples of working heights for varied tasks.

Shorten Reach Distance

Reach envelope is the term used to describe the area that can be reached in a safe position as the arm is moved around the shoulder or the forearm around the elbow.

The optimal reach envelope is close to the torso and is defined by movement of the forearm around the elbow while the elbows are comfortably at rest at the caregiver's sides. This is the area in which frequently performed work tasks should occur. The secondary reach envelope is defined by movement of the entire arm around the shoulder. This is the area in which infrequently performed work tasks should occur. Figure 3-10 illustrates the reach envelope concept.

Reduce Static Postures

Frequently changing position minimizes the effect of static postures and increases blood supply to muscles. For example, stand up and stretch or alternate between sitting and standing work tasks. See Figure 3-11 for an example of a standing workstation.

Reduce Forces and Loads

Reducing the physical effort required when performing tasks that involve forceful exertions, such as lifting, pushing, or grasping, may reduce the risk of injury.

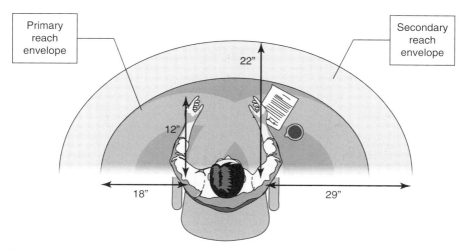

- Get closer to the work/equipment/tools
- Bring the work/equipment/tools to you
- Use a tool to reduce reach distance

FIGURE 3-10 Recommended reach envelope for frequently and infrequently performed tasks. *(Concept courtesy of Lynda Enos)*

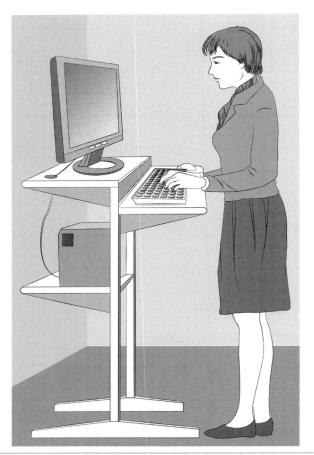

FIGURE 3-11 An example of a standing workstation.

Lifting Tasks

Although it is generally considered that many employees can safely lift up to a 50-pound object on an infrequent basis, this 50-pound lifting guideline does not apply if certain work design conditions exist. In addition, the guideline does not apply if a caregiver has suffered a back injury and has been advised by a physician to follow a specific restriction on the amount of weight that can be lifted, carried, pushed, or pulled. This lift limit also does not apply to manually lifting and moving clients. Refer to later chapters for more information about safe client handling.

Table 3-4 describes tips for moving loads safely.

If the load is too heavy or awkward, or is being handled below knee level or above shoulder height, good body mechanics may not be enough to

---

TABLE 3-4   Tips for Moving Loads Safely

"Body mechanics" refers to the way we move our bodies. Good body mechanics involve moving and positioning your body in such a way as to reduce physical stress on musculoskeletal structures. The following are tips to help maintain good body mechanics when lifting objects:

- Prepare the environment—ensure that the path to be traveled is clear of obstacles
- Plan your move—test the load and get help or equipment as necessary
- Mentally prepare
- Physically prepare
  - Use the body as a unit
  - Keep the load close to your body
  - Use a power grip if possible
  - Place feet shoulder-width apart to create a stable base
  - Lower your center of gravity
  - Keep your nose between your toes
  - Bend at the hips, not the waist
  - Point your toe where you want to go
  - Shift through your lower body
  - Never twist your back
  - Move the load steadily; avoid sudden motions

---

prevent acute or cumulative musculoskeletal disorders. Figure 3-12 illustrates the preferred height and distance from the body for lifting objects.

When possible, the caregiver should choose engineering controls such as mechanical equipment to lift and move objects. If equipment is not provided, the caregiver should get help from a coworker or coworkers to complete the task. It is important for the caregiver to remember that using good body mechanics alone cannot make an unsafe task into a safe one.

Carrying, Pushing, and Pulling

Using a cart is generally a good idea when carrying equipment and supplies that weigh more than 25 pounds and when travel distance is farther than 14 feet. Using both hands to push a cart or other equipment is safer than pulling. Some carts are designed to be moved from one end only, which is typically labeled, and will be difficult to steer or maneuver if pushed from the wrong end. (See Figure 3-13.) Prompt reporting of equipment problems and removing unsafe equipment from service are essential to caregiver and client safety.

Grip Force

Caregivers should select a tool that requires a power grip rather than a pinch grip to reduce forces associated with holding and manipulating tools and equipment. Maintaining neutral postures of the fingers, thumb, wrist, and

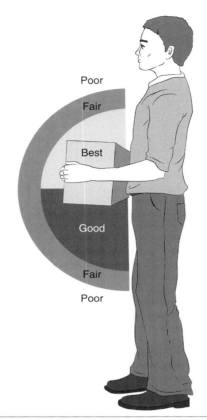

Poor

Fair

Best

Good

Fair

Poor

FIGURE 3-12 Preferred height and distance from the body for lifting objects.

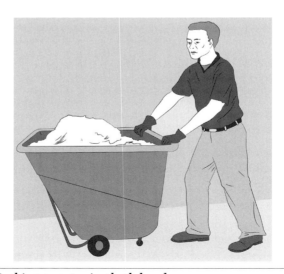

FIGURE 3-13 Pushing a cart using both hands.

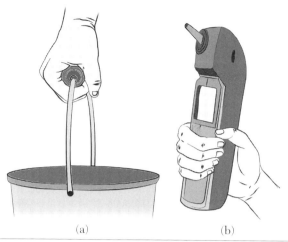

(a)   (b)

FIGURE 3-14 Proper equipment and tool design allows neutral posture of wrist and arm.

arm also reduces grip force. The caregiver should be able to use the tool in neutral postures relative to the work surface orientation. Tools and equipment that require repetitive, forceful use of one finger or thumb to operate should be avoided. Left-handed caregivers should request hand tools that are made for left-handed users. (See Figure 3-14.)

Minimize Contact Stress

Tools and equipment that create contact stress on the palm of the hand should be avoided. Avoid resting arms or wrists on worktable edges or leaning against work surfaces. Sharp edges can be rounded or padded to remove the contact stressor. (See Figure 3-15.) Allowing legs to hang from a chair unsupported can cause pressure on the back of the thigh, impeding circulation. The caregiver should use a footrest if the work surface is so high that feet cannot be positioned flat on the floor.

Reduce Repetition

By examining work tasks with coworkers, the work team may be able to generate ideas for good work practices and other controls to reduce exposure to repetitive awkward postures or motions to complete a task. Planning work and organizing work areas before beginning a task can reduce the number of motions used and reduce physical demands.

If different tasks require similar motions over a period of time, the caregiver should look for feasible ways to alternate use of different muscle groups by alternating job tasks.

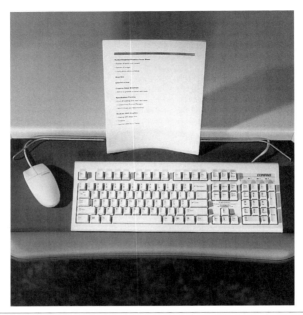

FIGURE 3-15 Sharp edges can be rounded or padded to remove the contact stressor.

Maintain a Comfortable Environment

Glare can be reduced by using blinds on windows, reducing lighting level (if practical), or using a hood or antiglare screen on the monitor.

Good housekeeping practices contribute to a safe and comfortable work environment, as does removing equipment and other items when they are no longer needed. A cluttered environment restricts access and impedes the ability to complete a task efficiently. Report hazards to your supervisor and area safety representative immediately.

Use Safe Work Practices

Safe work practices involve planning the task, assembling needed equipment and supplies, and organizing the work area before performing a task. Removing hazards from the environment, such as items that could cause you to slip or trip, and arranging furniture or equipment and tools to reduce reach distances and enable clear work access are also effective work-practice controls. Table 3-5 lists a three-step approach to help you remember to take time to prepare work tasks and use safe work practices.

Using Computers and Performing Data Entry

Computers used in health care may include desktop systems located at the nurses' station, portable systems mounted on roll-about workstations that

---

TABLE 3-5   Use Safe Work Practices

To facilitate safe work practices and reduce exposure risk to WRMSDs, take a few seconds to conduct a hazard or risk assessment before performing work tasks.

1. Always assess and prepare the environment
2. Get necessary equipment and help
3. Perform the task safely

---

can be moved from room to room, or laptop computers that can be taken into the home setting. See Figure 3-16 for an example of ergonomics controls for a desktop computer.

Chair

The caregiver should adjust chair height so that wrists are straight when using the keyboard and arms are approximately parallel to the floor. Legs should be at approximately right angles at hip, knee, and ankle. Use a footrest if feet are not supported on the floor. Remove any clutter under the workstation that may prevent enough room for legs and feet. Adjust the back of the chair so that your low back is supported and you are sitting in an upright position. Avoid leaning forward when performing data entry. The seat pan should support your legs and be deep enough to provide a 2- to 3-inch space between the front of the seat pan and the back of your knee. Some seat pans can adjust to reclining, forward, or flat angles. The seat pan should be padded, and have a rounded front edge. Chairs should have a five-point base of support. The caregiver should not use chairs that are broken or unstable. The chair should have adequate weight capacity to support the caregiver. Armrests should be used for support during data entry only if a neutral posture can be maintained; that is, the shoulders should be relaxed and not rolled forward or pushed up, and the elbows should be relaxed and close to the side of the body. Armrests should be removed if they interfere with work or increase reach distance by preventing the caregiver from moving close to the work surface or keyboard.

Keyboard

The keyboard should be positioned directly in front of the caregiver, allowing wrists and forearms to remain relatively straight. Some workstations may have a keyboard tray that allows height and angle adjustments. The keyboard tray should be large enough to accommodate other input devices such as a trackball or mouse. A wrist rest positioned in front of the keyboard can be used to support palms and wrists during rest periods from keying.

Sitting Diagram

This is the general diagram of the recommended sitting posture for computer users. It is important to change postures frequently when using a computer. Sitting for long periods can cause discomfort and muscle fatigue. To minimize fatigue:
- Take frequent microbreaks: stand up, walk around, or gently stretch.
- Change body position frequently by using adjustments on your chair. For example, place the back of the chair in a reclining position for a period of time; maintain correct alignment with monitor, keyboard, and mouse.
- Avoid leaning forward, slumping, or sitting on the edge of the chair.
- Give your eyes a break. Focus on a distant object, close your eyes regularly.
- Reduce repetitive motions by using shortcut commands and varying work tasks.

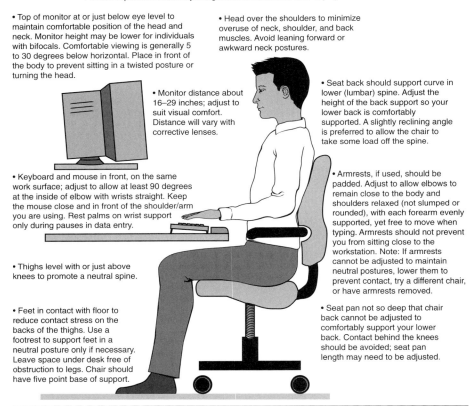

• Top of monitor at or just below eye level to maintain comfortable position of the head and neck. Monitor height may be lower for individuals with bifocals. Comfortable viewing is generally 5 to 30 degrees below horizontal. Place in front of the body to prevent sitting in a twisted posture or turning the head.

• Head over the shoulders to minimize overuse of neck, shoulder, and back muscles. Avoid leaning forward or awkward neck postures.

• Monitor distance about 16–29 inches; adjust to suit visual comfort. Distance will vary with corrective lenses.

• Seat back should support curve in lower (lumbar) spine. Adjust the height of the back support so your lower back is comfortably supported. A slightly reclining angle is preferred to allow the chair to take some load off the spine.

• Keyboard and mouse in front, on the same work surface; adjust to allow at least 90 degrees at the inside of elbow with wrists straight. Keep the mouse close and in front of the shoulder/arm you are using. Rest palms on wrist support only during pauses in data entry.

• Armrests, if used, should be padded. Adjust to allow elbows to remain close to the body and shoulders relaxed (not slumped or rounded), with each forearm evenly supported, yet free to move when typing. Armrests should not prevent you from sitting close to the workstation. Note: If armrests cannot be adjusted to maintain neutral postures, lower them to prevent contact, try a different chair, or have armrests removed.

• Thighs level with or just above knees to promote a neutral spine.

• Feet in contact with floor to reduce contact stress on the backs of the thighs. Use a footrest to support feet in a neutral posture only if necessary. Leave space under desk free of obstruction to legs. Chair should have five point base of support.

• Seat pan not so deep that chair back cannot be adjusted to comfortably support your lower back. Contact behind the knees should be avoided; seat pan length may need to be adjusted.

FIGURE 3-16 Using good body postures when working at a seated computer workstation.

The Mouse and Other Input or Pointing Devices

The caregiver should place the mouse or pointing device in the primary reach envelope at the same height as the keyboard, and to either side of it. (See Figure 3-17.) The arm should be close to the body. As with the keyboard, the hand, wrist, and forearm should be reasonably straight and positioned slightly above the mouse. A palm rest can help support the hand and

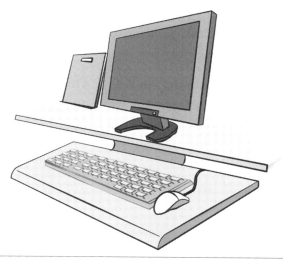

FIGURE 3-17 Mouse and keyboard should be on the same level, as shown. A good position for a document holder is also illustrated in this diagram.

keep the wrist straight. Other types of pointing devices include touch pads, trackballs, glide points, and mice designed for use by either hand.

Monitor

The monitor should be positioned directly in front of the caregiver. The top-most active line of text on the monitor screen should be at or slightly below eye level so that the caregiver's head is upright or tilted slightly forward, and comfortably balanced over the shoulders. The most frequently viewed area of the monitor should be about 15 degrees below eye level. The caregiver should avoid twisting the neck, bending it backward, or bending it more than a few degrees forward. If the workstation is used by several different caregivers, an easily adjustable monitor stand may be needed to allow each user to adjust it to meet individual needs. The distance between the screen and the eyes can be adjusted by moving the monitor forward or back until the viewing distance is visually comfortable. Caregivers with bifocal, trifocal, or progressive lenses may find viewing the monitor more comfortable if it is positioned lower to avoid tilting the head back to read through the bottom portion of the lens. Another option is to purchase a pair of glasses to use at the computer. (See Figure 3-18.)

Document Holders

A document holder should be stable and adjustable for height and angle of view. The caregiver should place the document holder close to the screen and at the same height and viewing distance to reduce eye, neck, or back strain when looking from screen to document. (Refer to Figure 3-17.)

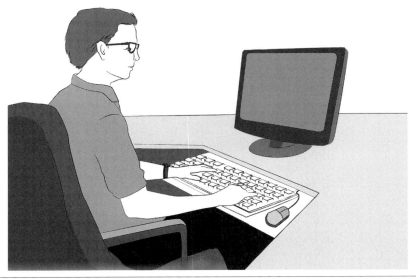

FIGURE 3-18 Monitor height may be lower for bifocal wearers.

Telephone and Other Equipment

The caregiver should arrange the workstation so that frequently used items, such as the telephone, are placed in the primary reach envelope to reduce reach distance. Headsets can increase productivity by making it easier to refer to files or to use the computer while on the phone.

Lighting and Glare

The workstation and monitor should be located away from and at right angles to windows and overhead light fixtures that create glare on the monitor screen. To reduce glare, close blinds on nearby windows or attach a visor hood to the monitor.

Standing Workstations

Standing workstations may be stationary, such as an order-entry station, or movable, such as a mobile computer cart. The principles for placement of equipment as described in previous sections also apply to standing workstations. Antifatigue matting may be provided to relieve pressure on the back and legs from prolonged standing.

Multi-User Workstations

It is likely that caregivers will share computer workstations with other caregivers and employees. It is important that multi-user workstations have features that allow all users to adjust the workstation to fit them comfortably.

In intensive care units and other settings where multiple monitors are viewed, the monitors should be placed close together and positioned so they can be viewed easily without using awkward neck postures.

Materials Handling in Storage Areas

Heavy and frequently used items should be stored just below waist height, at approximately 29 inches. Lighter-weight items that are frequently used should be stored between shoulder and knee height, and lightweight and rarely used items should be stored above shoulder height. (See Figure 3-19.) Whenever possible, avoid storing items overhead.

When available, the caregiver should use a cart with an adjustable platform or a platform that is level with the shelving. This allows items to be slid over from shelves and transported, rather than lifted and carried. Boxes or containers with handles or cutouts are easier to grip and hold. If items must be stored overhead, rather than reaching, use a stable step stool equipped with a handrail or a platform ladder. Shelves that are too deep require an

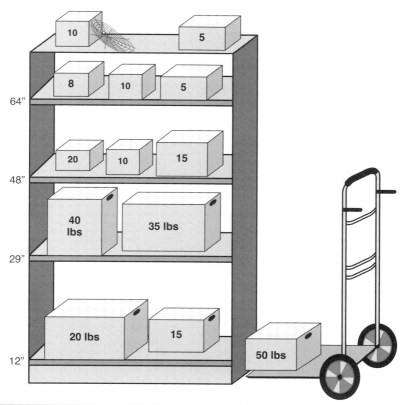

FIGURE 3-19 Recommended storage heights.

extended reach to retrieve items toward the back. Typically, approximately 20 inches is a good depth, unless a deeper shelf depth is needed to accommodate safe storage of larger items.

The caregiver should use a hand truck or get help to move heavy items stored on the floor. Labels listing approximate weight can be placed on items weighing more than 10 pounds to alert the caregiver to heavier loads that require assistance or equipment. Storing items close to the work area where they will be used also reduces carrying. Keep aisles clear and wide enough to allow access with mechanical lifting aids or carts.

Pushing Beds and Stretchers and Other Equipment

The caregiver should inspect equipment before use to ensure that it is in good working order. Many stretchers and wheelchairs have easy-to-access holders for oxygen and intravenous fluids, allowing access using neutral body postures. Carts with vertical handles allow caregivers of varied heights to grasp handles using the power grip, with the wrist in a neutral posture. (See Figure 3-20.) Motorized push–pull devices can be used to move beds, stretchers, and wheelchairs if there is enough hallway, elevator, and turning space in the facility. (See Figure 3-21.)

Preparing and Dispensing Medications

A mechanical pill crusher can be used if pills must be crushed. If crushed manually, use the minimum amount of force necessary to crush the pills, and

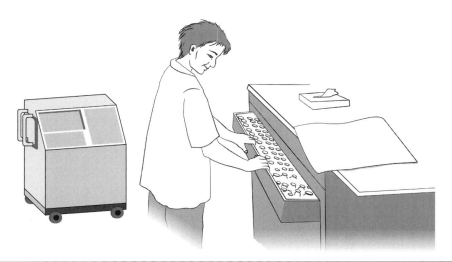

FIGURE 3-20 Examples of good cart design. *Vertical handles and large wheels reduce push force.*

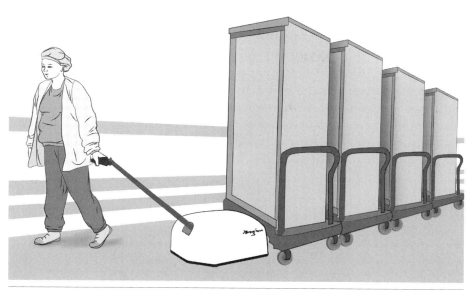

FIGURE 3-21 A motorized cart mover.

alternate hands used. Pharmaceutical guidelines prohibit crushing of certain medications. The caregiver should always check with the organization's medication administration guidelines to find out if a particular pill is safe to administer if crushed. The best solution may be to contact the client's physician and request the medication in liquid form if available.

Low-profile medication carts with easy-open drawers are recommended to accommodate hand height of shorter caregivers. Cart handles should be positioned to allow grasping with the wrist and hand in a neutral posture, with the wrists relatively straight. (See Figure 3-20.)

Handling Linen and Performing Laundry Tasks

Linen handling is often a shared responsibility between caregivers and housekeeping and laundry staff members.

Handling Bags of Soiled Laundry

Laundry bags should be changed when loosely filled, and more often if the linen is wet. Smaller bags may be an acceptable solution. Bags with handles provide for easier gripping. As with any load, it is a good idea for the caregiver to test the weight of the laundry bag before attempting to lift it. Rather than carrying the bags, caregivers should use a cart to move bags of soiled laundry to a laundry chute or soiled-linen cart. The caregiver should make an effort to avoid overfilling laundry carts, particularly those with removable sides.

Washing and Drying Laundry

False-bottomed laundry carts or carts with spring-loaded inserts can reduce forward bending by helping to keep the laundry at hip height. Washing machines and dryers should be installed so that the opening is between hip and elbow height. Bins used for unloading should be similar in height to the machine openings. Positioning them to one side helps to prevent reaching over bins or twisting to retrieve laundry. Reaching aids can be used to retrieve laundry from washing machines and dryers. If using top-loading washers, caregivers should handle small loads of laundry at one time. (See Figure 3-22.)

Folding and Sorting Laundry

Working-surface heights should be slightly below elbow height. Antifatigue matting and foot-rails or footrests may reduce caregiver fatigue in areas where prolonged standing is required.

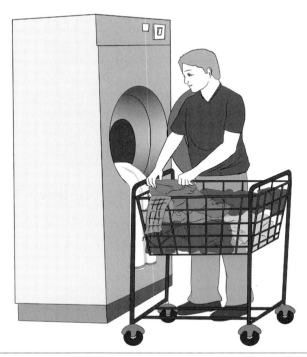

FIGURE 3-22 Laundry bins at the same height as washer and dryer openings reduce awkward postures.

Delivering and Stocking Clean Laundry

As previously mentioned, some carts are designed to be pushed or moved from one end. If there is a question with regard to this feature, the caregiver should ask the supervisor. For the safety of all, pushing a tall cart should be performed by two individuals if vision is obstructed. As mentioned above, carts should not be overfilled. Carts with handles are preferable. If the caregiver experiences difficulty pushing a cart, it should be reported. Motorized push-pull devices can be used to move laundry carts if there is enough hallway, elevator, and turning space in the facility. Refer to Figure 3-21 for an example of a motorized cart mover.

Housekeeping Tasks

Caregiver housekeeping tasks vary by health care setting. Good housekeeping is important to safety, and because of that, it should always be a team responsibility.

Room Cleaning

The caregiver can use telescoping and extension handles, hoses, and tools to reduce reaching. (See Figure 3-23.) Alternating the leading hand, keeping a loose, light grip rather than a tight, static grip, and using tools with padded nonslip handles can reduce caregiver fatigue when performing these tasks.

Cleaning surfaces in rooms is a task performed by caregivers in most health care settings. Trigger handles on spray bottles should be long enough for both the index and middle fingers to be used when squeezing. Squeezing cleaning cloths with wrists in a neutral posture minimizes hand wringing. Alternatively, using disposable cloths eliminates the wringing hazard. Knee pads can be used for frequent kneeling tasks. Carts should be used to transport supplies. Alternatively, the caregiver should carry only small quantities and weights of supplies.

The caregiver should change trash bags before they become overfull. Smaller trash and garbage containers hold less, thus reducing the force required to remove the full trash bags.

Cleaning Floors

Whenever possible, the caregiver should avoid lifting heavy buckets—for example, lifting a large, full bucket from a sink. By using a hose or similar device, buckets can be filled with water while on the floor or in position on the housekeeping cart. The caregiver should use buckets with wheels that roll easily and have functional brakes. Handles should be round and should be of sufficient diameter to allow the caregiver to grasp the handle with a power grip. Refer to Figure 3-14 for an illustration.

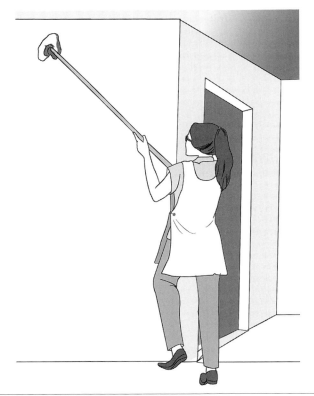

FIGURE 3-23 Tools with extended handles make cleaning jobs easier by reducing reach.

Mops with lightweight telescoping and adjustable-angle handles weigh less and may be easier to maneuver. Microfiber mops may be a suitable alternative to traditional mops. Wringer buckets with higher wringer attachments reduce forward bending. Longer, padded handles on the wringer require less force to wring mops, reduce contact stress on the hand and palm, and promote neutral posture of the wrist and arm. Swinging the mop in a horizontal "figure 8" direction allows the caregiver to complete the task with the elbows fairly close to the sides, essentially performing the task in the primary reach zone. Keeping safety in mind, the caregiver should mop one side of the floor at a time so there is always a dry surface for walking, and should consistently post warning signs when the floor is wet. Signs should be removed promptly when the floor is dry.

Vacuuming and Buffing Floors

Buffers with triggers long enough to accommodate at least the index and middle fingers, and vacuum cleaners and buffers with lightweight construction, adjustable handles, and easy-to-reach controls, help to reduce the use of force and awkward postures. The caregiver should use both hands when buffing and avoid using a tight grip. If vibration is a concern, vibration-damping materials and low-vibration buffers may be feasible controls.

Caregivers should avoid using a tight grip when vacuuming and should alternate hands to give forearm muscles a rest. Vacuum bags should be changed when half to three-quarters full.

Cleaning and Making Unoccupied Beds

When adjustable beds are available, taking the time to raise an adjustable bed to waist height before making it reduces awkward postures. Many facilities have electric adjustable beds. Once the bed is at the appropriate height, the caregiver should position the bed away from the wall, if possible, and should walk around the bed instead of reaching across.

Adjustable beds are typically not available in the home- or community-care environments. In these settings, good body mechanics is the primary control to minimize the risk of injury. Whenever possible, the caregiver should position supplies and the bed to minimize stooping or bending during bed-making tasks. Flipping a heavy mattress for cleaning is an awkward task and can be done more quickly and safely with two people. Lighter-weight mattresses are available, and are a good control.

Food Preparation and Serving

Working surfaces used for food preparation should be slightly below elbow height to allow for better visibility and control of the task. Food-grade antifatigue matting and foot-rails or footrests reduce fatigue in areas where prolonged standing is required, but may create trip hazards. Care should be taken in their selection. Floor surfaces should be kept clean and dry to prevent slipping.

Although it is a common practice in community-care settings, serving food by balancing a loaded tray on the palm of the hand with the wrist extended (bent backward) increases the risk of injury to both caregiver and client. Individual food trays should be carried one at a time, using both hands, or transported on a cart. If feasible, the caregiver should avoid storing trays on food-service cart shelves that are over shoulder height or below knee level.

EARLY RECOGNITION, REPORTING, AND TREATMENT OF WRMSDS

It is important that symptoms of WRMSDs be reported promptly. In general, the earlier the symptoms of musculoskeletal disorders are identified and treatment is initiated, the less likely a more serious disorder will develop. Early reporting increases the chances for successful treatment and rehabilitation.

Caregivers should be alert to tension, discomfort, or pain and take immediate action to relieve it.

If the caregiver suffers a WRMSD, the caregiver may be released to modified work if the employer has an early-return-to-work policy. The goal of return-to-work programs is to help injured workers make the transition back to regular work gradually and safely. Modified work typically involves only the parts of the job that can be done safely with minimal risk of injury or reinjury. Early-return-to-work programs benefit the employer and the caregiver.

The caregiver should request that an ergonomics evaluation be conducted of the work task that contributed to the WRMSD if one has not already been completed. Controls should be implemented to eliminate or minimize further caregiver exposure to risk factors or hazards.

C H A P T E R

4

SAFE CLIENT MOVEMENT AND HANDLING

INTRODUCTION

Moving and handling clients in the care environment has been performed manually for many years, but it is now widely recognized that this is a risky undertaking for both caregiver and client. A *lateral transfer* is a method of moving a client laterally, or horizontally, across a surface in a recumbent position—for example, from bed to stretcher. Traditional methods of performing lateral transfers or repositioning tasks such as moving a dependent client up in bed may place the client at risk by causing shear forces and friction. *Shear force* is action or stress resulting from applied forces, which causes, or is apt to cause, two adjacent internal body parts—for example, two skin layers—to move against each other. This stress is applied in opposite directions. *Friction* is a similar concept, but relates to the resistance to motion of the external tissue (i.e., skin) sliding in a parallel direction relative to the support surface (i.e., bed sheets). Shear force and friction may result in external tissue damage such as skin tears, friction burns, and pressure ulcers. These shear forces and friction may also increase caregiver forceful exertion, increasing risk of injury, especially to shoulders and back.

Clients and caregivers may also be at risk during other manual transfer tasks. Although it is not possible to eliminate hazards associated with client handling and movement, the research suggests that risk of these tasks can be greatly reduced through implementation of a comprehensive facility-specific program incorporating the proper use of carefully selected client-handling equipment and devices. This chapter provides basic information on safe client handling and movement strategies with examples of solutions. The information is not all-inclusive. The caregiver is encouraged to use reputable Web sites and other resources to seek current information on this topic, as it is a rapidly evolving area in client care.

RISK OF INJURY

Moving and handling clients typically requires awkward postures, presents physical demands, or force, beyond caregiver capability, and is performed frequently throughout a typical workday. As discussed in earlier chapters, awkward posture, excessive force, and repetition are musculoskeletal hazards, and each increases risk of injury.

For most client-handling tasks, the level of injury risk is typically related to:

- Dependency level of the client;

- Environmental assessment;

- Client-handling equipment options;

- Functional abilities of the caregiver and physical demands of the activity.

Dependency Level of Client

The client's **dependency level** describes the degree to which the client depends on others for activities of daily living, including the ability to move. One method of determining dependency levels uses three dependency level categories, based on client assessment:

1. **Independent**—client performs task safely, with or without staff assistance, with or without assistive devices.

2. **Partial assist**—client requires no more help than standby, cueing, or coaxing, or caregiver is required to lift no more than 35 pounds of a client's weight.

3. **Dependent**—client requires caregiver to lift more than 35 pounds of the client's weight, or the amount of assistance needed is unpredictable. (In this case assistive devices should be used.)

Environmental Assessment

Room design and the type of furniture in the room can contribute to awkward postures. A good environmental assessment extends outside the client room and should involve the entire travel path of the client.

Client-Handling Equipment Options

Appropriate, safe equipment, as an engineering control, is an essential element of a safe client movement and handling program. Proper selection of equipment is critical. Choice of equipment or device should be based on safety and equipment design, and on the individual client's functional strength and abilities, medical and cognitive status, and rehabilitative care plan.

Health care organizations should have guidelines to ensure that each product considered for purchase is carefully evaluated for safety and to confirm that it is an appropriate match for the client-care environment and population. Regular, thorough, ongoing training on safe operation and use of each device, and clear policies and procedures related to its use and care, is of critical importance.

Detailed guidance related to specific client-handling equipment and device decisions is beyond the scope of this guide, and specific questions should be directed to a safety professional with special training in this area. The following paragraphs describe examples of various technological solutions available to make client movement and handling safer. These illustrations and discussion, and other illustrations and discussions in this chapter, are not product endorsements, but rather are intended to show examples of equipment types or categories available.

Floor-Based Lifts (Portable Lifts)

Traditionally, moving a client from a chair or wheelchair to bed has been performed either manually or using a Hoyer lift (Hoyer is not a type of lift; rather, it is a brand). The Hoyer lift operates by a hydraulic pump mechanism, which, when engaged, raises and lowers the client by manually pumping the handle up and down. The base legs are operated manually as well.

The hydraulic Hoyer lift is one example of a **floor-based lift device.** A floor-based lift device is a portable device designed to lift and carry a client from one place to another (bed to chair). Most whole-body floor-based lift devices are battery powered and come in a variety of brands and styles, produced by an array of manufacturers. A sling is placed under or around the client, depending on the task, and secured to a spreader bar or crossbar on the lift. A **sling** is a device, usually made of sturdy fabric, designed for use with mechanical lifting equipment to temporarily suspend a body or body part in order to perform a client-handling task. Slings are designed for specific purposes, and some can be left under the client. A sling should be inspected for wear and other defects on a regular basis to ensure safety of both client and caregiver. By using a powered device, raising and lowering a client can be done by simply pressing a button on a control unit, which is faster and easier, and leaves the caregiver free to observe the client in the lift as well as the surrounding environment. In some models, there is also the capability to open and close the base of the unit by powered means. A dynamic positioning feature available on some lifts enables the caregiver to mechanically adjust the range of recline (or tilt) for clients who have to maintain a specific sitting posture during the transfer. Clients with respiratory compromise have reported feeling more comfortable when this feature is used during transfers. These features reduce injury risk as compared with the nonpowered lift, and they make the lift safer and more comfortable for the client and caregiver.

Powered Transport Devices

A **powered transport device** is typically a battery-operated motorized unit operated by the caregiver to move large or heavy wheeled objects such as occupied beds, gurneys, and wheelchairs. The caregiver activates the motor and steers the unit to the desired location. Often the device is a detachable, independent unit that can be attached to a bed, gurney, or wheelchair. In other cases, the powered transport mechanism is integrated, such as powered beds. The caregiver unplugs the bed from the wall and presses a button on the handles at the head of the bed to propel the bed forward. (See Figures 4-1 and 4-2.)

Electric Height-Adjustable Beds

Some brands of electric beds, called "fast" electric beds, are designed to change height at a much faster rate of speed than older electric beds, generally in approximately 20 to 25 seconds. These beds can be lowered nearly to floor level and are widely used in long-term care settings. Although these beds typically have a weight capacity of up to 500 pounds, specially designed beds are also available with higher weight capacity and the ability to expand in width to accommodate larger clients. (See Figure 4-3.)

Wheelchair Mover

A wheelchair mover is a battery-operated device that attaches to any standard wheelchair, propelling it forward by simply pushing or pulling a lever. An example is provided in Figure 4-1.

Assistive Devices for Repositioning in Bed

Repositioning tasks can often be performed more safely and efficiently with the use of a **friction-reducing device,** typically made of a foldable fabric

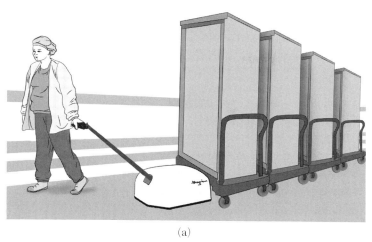

(a)

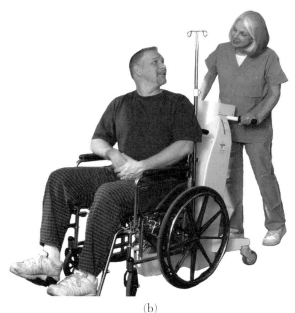

(b)

FIGURE 4-1 Examples of detachable powered transport devices: (a) powered transport devices can be used to pull laundry and dietary carts; (b) specially designed devices latch firmly to wheelchairs to reduce the effort needed to move the client. (*Courtesy of Dane Technologies, Inc.*)

or similar material with a slippery surface. The device is placed under the client and slides easily over itself or over the bedding, depending on the product design, making the task easier and safer. Some are stitched together along one side in a tube configuration, with slippery surfaces on the inside against each other. Still others have a gel substance contained within

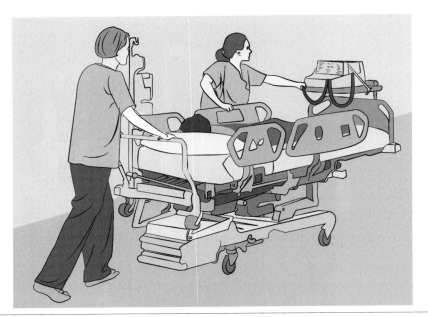

FIGURE 4-2 A powered bed.

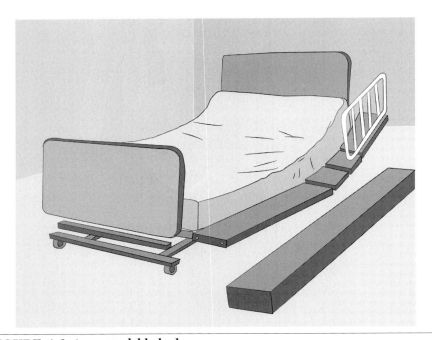

FIGURE 4-3 An expandable bed.

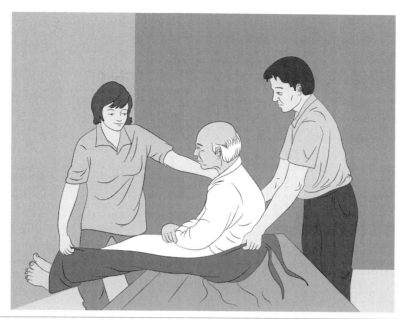

FIGURE 4-4 Friction-reducing repositioning device.

two fabric layers; the gel provides the slipperiness needed to reduce the force of the task. (See Figure 4-4.)

Other options for repositioning in bed include bed handles, **bed ladders,** bed rails, or ceiling lifts. A bed ladder is a ladder-like device that attaches to the foot of the bed. Clients grasp each rung and "climb" until they have reached a seated position. For dependent clients, a good option is a ceiling-mounted whole body lift with a sling. The **ceiling-mounted lift** works by suspending the client in a sling from a track, or rail, which is securely mounted to the ceiling or wall.

Functional Abilities of the Caregiver and Physical Demands of the Activity

Functional ability includes an individual's tolerance and ability to sit or stand or to lift, carry, push, or pull an object. It also includes range of movement, flexibility, endurance, and strength. If a task exceeds the caregiver's functional ability, it may place both caregiver and client at risk of injury.

Body Parts at High Risk in Client Movement and Handling

Specific risks to client body parts during manual client-handling tasks include bruising or skin tears and friction burns. Risk of hip fracture or head injury may be increased for clients who may suddenly and unpredictably lose their ability to stand independently during a transfer task.

Client-handling tasks impose high stresses on the caregiver's low back, neck, shoulders, and wrists. Physical stresses inflicted by client movement and handling tasks differ from stresses inflicted by lifting a box or other object. Multiple awkward postures occur simultaneously in these tasks, including any combination of horizontal reaching, bending at the waist, twisting of the spine, grasping with hands, lifting, pulling or pushing, and sustained gripping with one or both hands.

USING THE HIERARCHY OF CONTROLS TO REDUCE THE RISK OF CLIENT MOVEMENT AND HANDLING TASKS

Equipment and devices used for client movement and handling are considered engineering controls. It is not possible to eliminate client movement and handling tasks in health care. However, consistent and conscientious selection, use, and maintenance of appropriate engineering controls is second in effectiveness only to hazard elimination in reducing injury risk associated with these tasks.

Many health care facilities have developed comprehensive ergonomics programs that serve as administrative controls to guide safe client handling work practices. These programs typically include policies, procedures, and training necessary for the caregiver to know when a certain piece of equipment is appropriate and how to use the equipment safely. Risk assessment is an administrative control that aids in program development and prioritizing interventions.

The following paragraphs provide additional discussion related to how certain controls can be used in combination to reduce risk when performing specific client movement and handling tasks.

Lateral Transfers

Use of a lateral transfer device has been shown to reduce pull forces related to this task significantly. Examples of lateral-transfer devices are provided in the following paragraphs.

Air-Assisted Lateral-Transfer Devices

Use of an **air-assisted lateral-transfer device** reduces the friction and shear forces normally present during the transfer. The device is a flexible mattress placed under the client. Air flows through perforations on the bottom surface of the mattress from a portable air supply, forming a cushion of

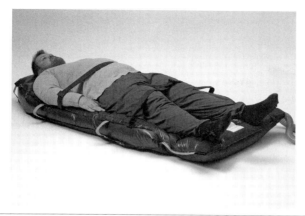

FIGURE 4-5 Air-assisted lateral-transfer device.

air. The client rests on the mattress, which is moved on this cushion of air, allowing staff members to position the client with much less effort. This method of transfer can be much more comfortable and safer for the client, as well, and is particularly suitable when performing lateral transfers involving clients with special medical conditions, such as pressure ulcers. This is an example of a product that benefits the caregiver while enhancing the quality of care for the dependent client. (See Figure 4-5.)

Mechanical Lateral-Transfer Devices

Mechanical lateral-transfer devices transfer the load of the lateral transfer to equipment designed for this purpose. These transfer aids reduce caregiver risk by reducing shoulder force, awkward lumbar posture, and sustained wrist activity (from pulling the drawsheet). They reduce client risk by reducing shear force and friction.

There are only a few mechanical transfer devices available that improve safety in this way. One is a height-adjustable stretcher with a hand crank that is used to transfer a client on and off the stretcher. Another type of mechanical lateral-transfer aid works by attaching two straps from the device to a metal rod that is rolled in the drawsheet to form an attachment point. The client lies on this sheet. A button is then depressed and the straps retract, pulling the client over to the destination surface. Figure 4-6 shows such a device.

Friction-Reducing Devices

There are a number of friction-reducing devices designed for lateral transfers. These are similar to other friction-reducing devices. Handles along the long side are a useful feature in reducing the amount of forward reach often required during lateral transfer tasks.

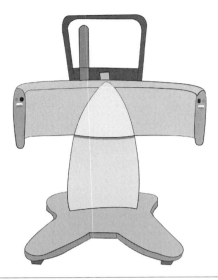

FIGURE 4-6 Mechanical lateral-transfer aid.

Bed-to-Chair Transfer

Examples of devices that can be used to do this task more easily and safely are provided in the following paragraphs.

Portable Floor-Based Lift

A powered mechanical lift works with use of a sling that is placed under or around the client, a spreader bar to which the sling connects, and a portable floor-based unit. It is operated by pressing a button to raise and lower the client. These portable units have adjustable legs that enable maneuvering around furniture. Many of these units can lift a client from the floor, some can be used to assist a client from a seated position in a vehicle, and some also can be used as ambulation aids. These lifts can be purchased with an integrated scale or a scale attachment for ease in obtaining client weight. Figure 4-7 shows a powered portable floor-based lift.

Ceiling Lifts

Ceiling lifts are beneficial in a variety of client-care tasks, including transferring clients from bed to chair, floor to bed or chair, or toilet to bed. They can be purchased with scale attachments for ease in obtaining client weight. Specially designed slings allow these lifts to be used for repositioning and to suspend an extremity, such as a leg, during wound care. They are also used as an ambulation aid. This technology works by suspending the client in a sling from a track or rail that is securely bolted to the ceiling or wall. At the

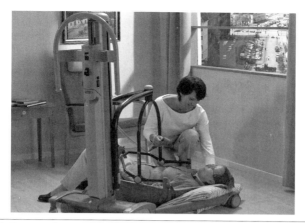

FIGURE 4-7 Powered portable floor-based lift. *(Courtesy of ARJO, Inc., Roselle, IL)*

time of this writing, there are basically two types of tracks available, a single or dedicated track and an X-Y track. The first track type allows the client to be moved only along the area that the track covers (i.e., in a straight path). The second type of track has more versatility because the coverage area is larger, and this design allows the client to be moved around the room. Ceiling track systems take up no floor space, require less force to operate than a floor-based lift, and do not have to be moved into the room to be used. Use of a ceiling lift eliminates the need to maneuver over uneven floor surfaces and around furniture as could be required with use of a floor-based lift. See Figure 4-8 for examples.

Sit-to-Stand (Stand-up) Lifts

A sit-to-stand lift is a device that can be used effectively to transfer clients who are cooperative and able to bear weight, but may have difficulty in standing up or are unsteady when ambulating. This type of lift typically has a sling that wraps around the upper abdomen below the axilla, and some models add straps under the thighs, as well. Once the sling is applied, the client presses the knees and the anterior lower legs against pads on the lower part of the lift while grasping handles with both hands. The lift raises the client from a seated position into a semi-standing position. The caregiver can then roll the client to the commode for toileting or to a chair, and lower the client into position. See Figure 4-8 for an example. Some sit-to-stand models apply excessive pressure under the axilla, and this is an important selection consideration.

Integrated Bed Systems

An **integrated bed system** refers to a bed with many integrated features, many of which can be used to reduce manual client handling. Such integrated

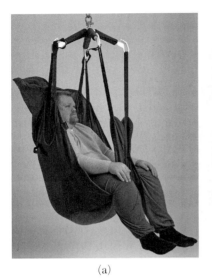

(a)

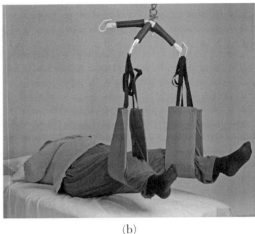

(b)

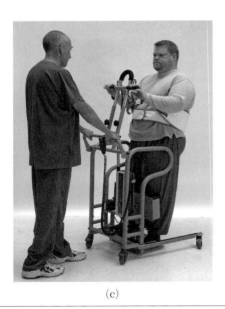

(c)

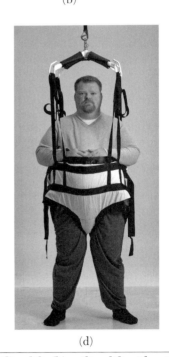

(d)

FIGURE 4-8 Examples of lifts: **(a) bariatric ceiling lift; (b) ceiling lift with extremity sling; (c) sit-to-stand lift; (d) bariatric walking sling.** *(Courtesy of Alpha Modalities, Seattle, WA)*

features include **chair positioning,** in which the bed converts to a chair-like configuration, percussion and vibration, and lateral rotation therapy. Currently, such specialized beds are available and used widely in critical-care and other intensive-care units to facilitate improved quality of care and save time for staff.

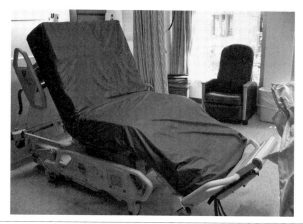

FIGURE 4-10 Chair positioning in integrated bed system. *(Courtesy of Kaiser-Permanente, NW Region, Kaiser Sunnyside Medical Center, Clackamas, OR)*

Chair positioning is important in rehabilitation; this task can be made easier by pressing a button and using the mechanical shearless pivot feature of the bed to assist a client from a lying to a sitting position (see Figure 4-10). This type of bed is especially beneficial for **bariatric clients,** for whom weights can exceed 400 pounds and body mass presents unique client-care challenges. Typically, bariatric clients are those with health, mobility, and environmental access limitations due to physical size.

BARIATRIC CARE

Obesity is a term used to describe a range of weight greater than that which is typically thought to be healthy. Exact definitions vary, but a body mass index of 30 or greater is generally considered **obese.**

For adults, overweight and obesity ranges are determined by a number called the **body mass index (BMI).** The BMI is calculated from a person's weight and height and generally provides a reliable indicator of body fat. It is commonly used to screen for weight categories that may lead to health problems and challenges to performing activities of daily living. As Table 4-1 illustrates, an adult who has a BMI between 25 and 29.9 is considered overweight, and an adult who has a BMI of 30 or higher is considered obese.

Caring for the bariatric client places caregivers at an increased risk of injury because of the excessive mass of the client and the multiple medical conditions associated with obesity. A bariatric client can be described as an individual with health limitations, mobility difficulties, or environmental access challenges related to physical size. The Veterans Affairs Patient Safety Center of Inquiry recommends implementing bariatric care guidelines

TABLE 4-1   Body Mass Index for Adults

Body Mass Index	Weight Status
Less than 18.5	Underweight
18.5–24.9	Normal
25.0–29.9	Overweight
30.0 and over	Obese

Adapted from BMI—Body Mass Index: BMI for Adults, Centers for Disease Control and Prevention, http://www.cdc.gov/nccdphp/dnpa/bmi/bmi-adult.htm

when the BMI exceeds 50, but for safety reasons, recommends that bariatric care guidelines be consistently instituted when a client exceeds the weight limit or size of standard existing equipment (approximately 300 pounds), regardless of BMI.

It is critical to client and caregiver safety to evaluate each client and establish whether special equipment is needed. For facilities that do not keep this specialized equipment on hand, a plan should be in place to obtain this equipment on short notice.

Integrated bed systems with specialty mattresses such as lateral-rotation features designed for bariatric clients may reduce risk factors associated with some care tasks. The caregiver can use the lateral-rotation feature to assist in turning the client to the side to complete client-care tasks, such as placing a bariatric sling in preparation for a lifting task with an expanded-capacity, or bariatric, lift appropriate to the client. Beds should be selected based on client weight and size. Choosing an expanded-capacity bed that is too wide places the caregiver at risk of injury because of excessive reaching distance. Expanded-capacity lifts may be ceiling mounted or floor based, but in either case it is imperative that the weight capacity be sufficient for the client. Bariatric convertible chairs may prove useful when transporting bariatric clients to procedures, as they allow the chair to change to multiple positions (seated, reclined, or flat). Some of these units have integrated battery-operated motors to aid transport. For units not equipped with powered transport features, a detachable powered transport device should be considered to reduce caregiver risk and preserve client dignity.

Client Dignity and Sensitivity

Caring for the bariatric client may present unique challenges. One way to approach care for bariatric clients that can promote dignity and sensitivity is by the using the acronym "EC" to designate oversized, expanded-weight capacity equipment—for example, the "EC commode." Safety professionals from the Mayo Clinic developed this idea, and have been using it success-fully for several years. The "EC" label allows staff to communicate with one another when special bariatric equipment is needed for client safety but reduces the chances of inadvertent and possibly hurtful use of terms such as "Big Boy Wheelchair." Another effective way to preserve dignity is to pre-pare prior to the arrival of a bariatric client whenever possible. A special bariatric admission process and bariatric policy may prove useful as an administrative control to foster communication, guide work practices, and standardize care for this special client population.

USING THE PATIENT SAFETY CENTER OF INQUIRY ASSESSMENT AND CARE-PLANNING FORM AND ALGORITHMS

Assessment criteria, care plans, and **algorithms** have been developed by the Department of Veterans Affairs Veterans Integrated Service Network 8 (VISN 8) Patient Safety Center of Inquiry to guide caregivers in considering client characteristics when selecting equipment and techniques for client handling and movement tasks. An algorithm is a step-by-step protocol used for managing health care challenges and changing conditions. These algorithms are presented later in this section.

The caregiver is reminded that the assessment criteria and algorithms are guidelines, and are appropriate for use only in care environments where the organization has invested in the necessary equipment and devices needed for safe client handling and movement. As with any guide-lines, these are intended to serve as an aid to critical clinical decision mak-ing, not as a substitute for the sound professional judgment so vital to the safety of clients and caregivers. It is prudent, as it is with any guideline, to seek information from additional reliable sources and to critically review the information to ensure that it is the most current and remains clinically sound and relevant.

Assessment and Planning Process for Safe Client Handling and Movement

Each care setting will have a unique approach to the assessment of safe client handling and movement and care planning, based on client population and level of care. Table 4-2 lists examples of important assess-ment criteria and key points for caregivers to consider when selecting equipment and techniques based on the client's unique characteristics and needs.

TABLE 4-2   Caregiver Considerations for Client-Centered Equipment Selection for Safe Client Handling and Movement

Key Points for Caregivers

Assess the patient.

Assess the area.

Decide on equipment.

Know how to use equipment.

Plan lift, and communicate with staff and patient.

Work together, including actions of more than one caregiver as well as the patient.

Have the right equipment available, in good working order, and conveniently located.

Key Assessment Criteria

Ability of the patient to provide assistance

Ability of the patient to bear weight

Upper extremity strength of the patient

Ability of the patient to consistently cooperate and follow instructions

Patient height and weight

Special circumstances likely to affect transfer or repositioning tasks, such as abdominal wounds, contractures, or presence of tubes, etc.

Specific physician orders or physical therapy recommendations that relate to transferring or repositioning patients (e.g., a patient with a knee or hip replacement may need a specific order or recommendation to maintain the correct angle of hip or knee flexion during transfer)

Source: *Patient care ergonomics resource guide: Safe patient handling and movement,* August, 2005, Tampa, FL: Patient Safety Center of Inquiry.

Assessment Criteria and Care-Planning Form for Safe Client Handling and Movement

The form shown in Figure 4-11 is a standardized form that the care team can complete collaboratively and captures key client-specific assessment information pertinent to choosing the safest method to move the client. The Key Assessment Criteria are also listed in Table 4-2. Note that client height and weight are listed. For the purposes of this assessment process, because of the weight capacity of most standardized equipment, a client weighing 300 pounds and having a BMI over 50 has been established as the defining criterion for a bariatric client.

Using the Safe Client Handling Algorithms

Once the Key Assessment Criteria have been logged onto the form, the care team reviews the information and consults the appropriate set of algorithms (bariatric or not) to determine the safest method of lifting and moving this specific client. The team then considers the unit or facility

Assessment Criteria and Care Plan for Safe Patient Handling and Movement

I. **Patient's Level of Assistance:**

_____ Independent— Patient performs task safely, with or without staff assistance, with or without assistive devices.

_____ Partial Assist—Patient requires no more help than stand-by, cueing, or coaxing, or caregiver is required to lift no more than 35 pounds of a patient's weight.

_____ Dependent—Patient requires nurse to lift more than 35 pounds of the patient's weight, or is unpredictable in the amount of assistance offered. In this case assistive devices should be used.

An assessment should be made prior to each task if the patient has varying level of ability to assist due to medical reasons, fatigue, medications, etc. When in doubt, assume the patient cannot assist with the transfer/repositioning.

II. **Weight Bearing Capability**   III. **Bi-Lateral Upper Extremity Strength**

_____ Full   _____ Yes
_____ Partial   _____ No
_____ None

IV. **Patient's level of cooperation and comprehension:**

_____ Cooperative — may need prompting; able to follow simple commands.

_____ Unpredictable or varies (patient whose behavior changes frequently should be considered as "unpredictable"), not cooperative, or unable to follow simple commands.

V. **Weight:** _____ **Height:** _____

Body Mass Index (BMI) [needed if patient's weight is over 300][1]: _____

If BMI exceeds 50, institute Bariatric Algorithms

The presence of the following conditions are likely to affect the transfer/repositioning process and should be considered when identifying equipment and technique needed to move the patient.

VI. **Check applicable conditions likely to affect transfer/repositioning techniques.**

_____ Hip/Knee/Shoulder Replacements   _____ Respiratory/Cardiac Compromise   _____ Fractures
_____ History of Falls   _____ Wounds Affecting Transfer/Positioning _____ Splints/Traction
_____ Paralysis/Paresis   _____ Amputation   _____ Severe Osteoporosis
_____ Unstable Spine   _____ Urinary/Fecal Stoma   _____ Severe Pain/Discomfort
_____ Severe Edema   _____ Contractures/Spasms   _____ Postural Hypotension
_____ Very Fragile Skin   _____ Tubes (IV, Chest, etc.)

Comments:_____
_____
_____

VII. Care Plan:			
Algorithm	Task	Equipment/ Assistive Device	# Staff
1	Transfer To and From: Bed to Chair, Chair To Toilet, Chair to Chair, or Car to Chair		
2	Lateral Transfer To and From: Bed to Stretcher, Trolley		
3	Transfer To and From: Chair to Stretcher, or Chair to Exam Table		
4	Reposition in Bed: Side-to-Side, Up in Bed		
5	Reposition in Chair: Wheelchair and Dependency Chair		
6	Transfer Patient Up from the Floor		
Bariatric 1	Bariatric Transfer To and From: Bed to Chair, Chair to Toilet, or Chair to Chair		
Bariatric 2	Bariatric Lateral Transfer To and From: Bed to Stretcher or Trolley		
Bariatric 3	Bariatric Reposition in Bed: Side-to-Side, Up in Bed		
Bariatric 4	Bariatric Reposition in Chair: Wheelchair, Chair or Dependency Chair		
Bariatric 5	Patient Handling Tasks Requiring Access to Body Parts (Limb, Abdominal Mass, Gluteal Area)		
Bariatric 6	Bariatric Transporting (Stretcher)		
Bariatric 7	Bariatric Toileting Tasks		

Sling Type: Seated_____   Seated (Amputation)_____   Standing_____   Supine_____   Ambulation_____   Limb Support_____

Sling Size: _____

Signature: _____   **Date:** _____

[1]If patient's weight is over 300 pounds, the BMI is needed. For Online BMI table and calculator see:
http://www.nhlbi.nih.gov/guidelines/obesity/bmi_tbl.htm

FIGURE 4-11 Example of assessment criteria and care-planning form for safe client handling and movement. *(Courtesy of the VISN 8 Patient Safety Center of Inquiry, Tampa, FL)*

equipment inventory, makes arrangements to obtain needed equipment not on hand, and records the appropriate device to be used for each of the client-handling tasks listed on the care plan. The boxes within the algorithm and the accompanying text provide tips and safety checks that should be observed prior to and during the transfer, and those can be noted on the form, as well. The process requires ongoing communication, teamwork, collaboration, and professional judgment and is expected to result in a safer environment for client and caregiver. Algorithms for a client of normal weight are provided in Figure 4-12, and algorithms for a bariatric client are provided in Figure 4-13.

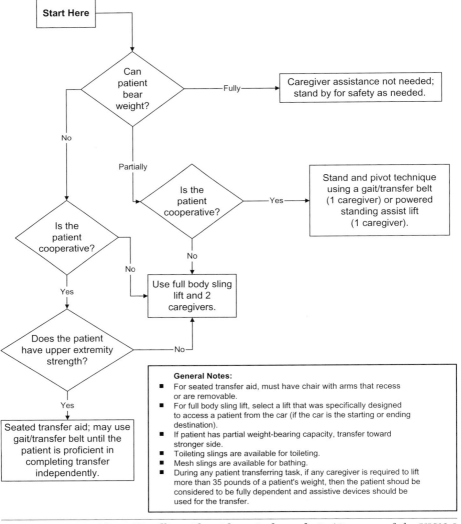

Algorithm 1: Transfer to and from: Bed to Chair, Chair to Toilet, Chair to Chair, or Car to Chair
Last rev. 8/22/06

FIGURE 4-12 Client-Handling Algorithms 1 through 6. (*Courtesy of the VISN 8 Patient Safety Center of Inquiry, Tampa, FL*)

Algorithm 2: Lateral Transfer to and from: Bed to Stretcher, Trolley
Last rev. 4/1/05

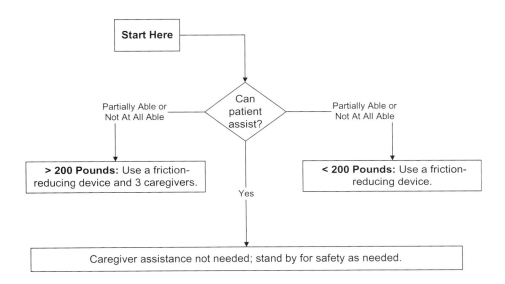

Start Here

Can patient assist?

Partially Able or Not At All Able

Partially Able or Not At All Able

> 200 Pounds: Use a friction-reducing device and 3 caregivers.

< 200 Pounds: Use a friction-reducing device.

Yes

Caregiver assistance not needed; stand by for safety as needed.

General Notes:
- Surfaces should be even for all lateral patient moves.
- For patients with Stage III or IV pressure ulcers, care must be taken to avoid shearing force.
- During any patient transferring task, if any caregiver is required to lift more than 35 pounds of a patient's weight, then the patient should be considered to be fully dependent and assistive devices should be used for the transfer.

FIGURE 4-12 *(continued)*

Algorithm 3: Transfer to and from: Chair to Stretcher or Chair to Exam Table
Last rev. 4/1/05

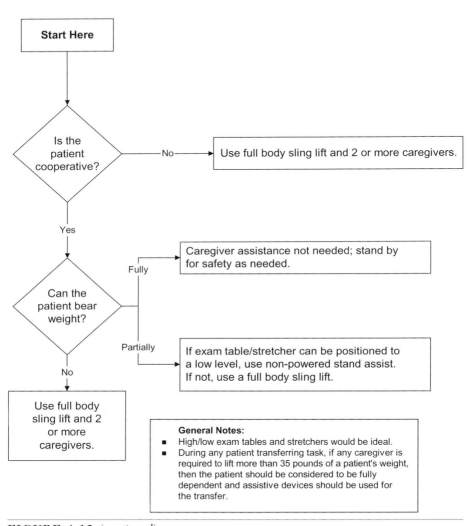

FIGURE 4-12 *(continued)*

Algorithm 4: Reposition in Bed: Side to Side, Up in Bed
Last rev. 4/1/05

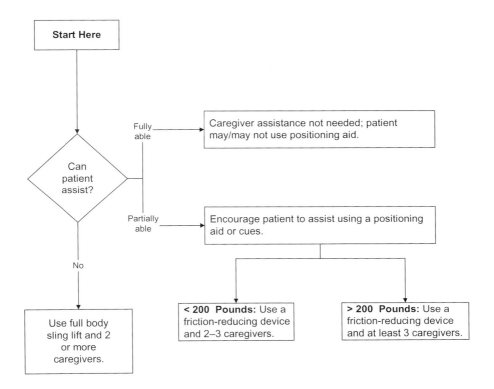

General Notes:
- This is not a one-person task: DO NOT PULL FROM HEAD OF BED.
- When pulling a patient up in bed, the bed should be flat or in a Trendelenburg position (when tolerated) to aid in gravity, with the side rail down.
- For patients with Stage III or IV pressure ulcers, care should be taken to avoid shearing force.
- The height of the bed should be appropriate for staff safety (at the elbows).
- If the patient can assist when repositioning "up in bed," ask the patient to flex the knees and push on the count of three.
- During any patient-handling task, if the caregiver is required to lift more than 35 pounds of a patient's weight, then the patient should be considered to be fully dependent and assistive devices should be used.

FIGURE 4-12 *(continued)*

Algorithm 5: Reposition in Chair: Wheelchair and Dependency Chair
Last rev. 8/23/05

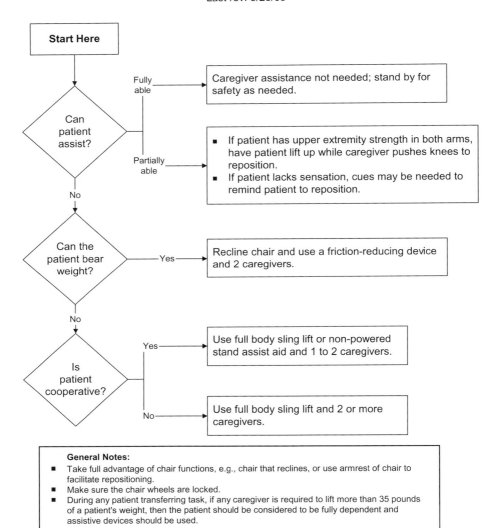

General Notes:
- Take full advantage of chair functions, e.g., chair that reclines, or use armrest of chair to facilitate repositioning.
- Make sure the chair wheels are locked.
- During any patient transferring task, if any caregiver is required to lift more than 35 pounds of a patient's weight, then the patient should be considered to be fully dependent and assistive devices should be used.

FIGURE 4-12 (*continued*)

Algorithm 6: Transfer a Patient Up from the Floor
Last rev. 4/1/05

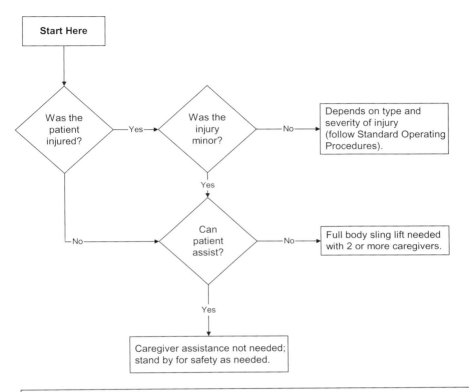

General Notes:
- Use full body sling lift that goes all the way down to the floor (most of the newer models are capable of this).
- During any patient transferring task, if any caregiver is required to lift more than 35 pounds of a patient's weight then the patient should be considered to be fully dependent and assistive devices should be used.

FIGURE 4-12 *(continued)*

Bariatric Algorithm 1: Bariatric Transfer to and from: Bed and Chair, Chair and Toilet, or Chair and Chair

rev. 8/23/06

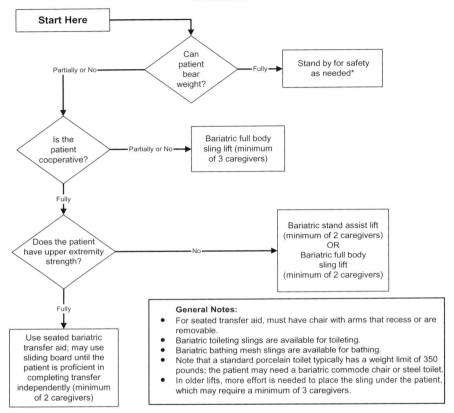

General Notes:
- For seated transfer aid, must have chair with arms that recess or are removable.
- Bariatric toileting slings are available for toileting.
- Bariatric bathing mesh slings are available for bathing.
- Note that a standard porcelain toilet typically has a weight limit of 350 pounds; the patient may need a bariatric commode chair or steel toilet.
- In older lifts, more effort is needed to place the sling under the patient, which may require a minimum of 3 caregivers.

* "Stand by for safety." In most cases, if a bariatric patient is about to fall, there is very little that the caregiver can do to prevent the fall. The caregiver should be prepared to move any items out of the way that could cause injury, try to protect the patient's head from striking any objects or the floor, and seek assistance as needed once the person has fallen.
- If patient has partial weight-bearing capability, transfer toward stronger side.
- Consider using an abdominal binder if the patient's abdomen impairs a patient-handling task.
- Assure equipment used meets weight requirements. Standard equipment is generally limited to 250–350 pounds. Facilities should apply a sticker to all bariatric equipment with "EC" (for expanded capacity) and a space for the manufacturer's rated weight capacity for that particular equipment model.
- Identify a leader when performing tasks with multiple caregivers. This will assure that the task is synchronized for increased safety of the health care provider and the patient.
- During any patient transferring task, if any caregiver is required to lift more than 35 pounds of a patient's weight, then the patient should be considered to be fully dependent and assistive devices should be used for the transfer.

FIGURE 4-13 Bariatric Client-Handling Algorithms 1 through 7. *(Courtesy of the VISN 8 Patient Safety Center of Inquiry, Tampa, FL)*

Bariatric Algorithm 2: Bariatric Lateral Transfer to and from: Bed, Stretcher, or Trolley
rev. 1/3/06

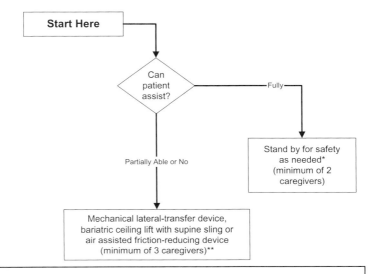

General Notes:
- The destination surface should be about 1/2" lower for all lateral patient moves.
- Avoid shearing force.
- Make sure bed is the right width, so excessive reaching by caregiver is not required.
- Lateral transfers should not be used with specialty beds that interfere with the transfer. In this case, use a bariatric ceiling lift with supine sling.
- Ensure bed or stretcher doesn't move with the weight of the patient transferring.
- ** Use a bariatric stretcher or trolley if patient exceeds weight capacity of traditional equipment.

---

* "Stand by for safety." In most cases, if a bariatric patient is about to fall, there is very little that the caregiver can do to prevent the fall. The caregiver should be prepared to move any items out of the way that could cause injury, try to protect the patient's head from striking any objects or the floor, and seek assistance as needed once the person has fallen.

* Assure equipment used meets weight requirements. Standard equipment is generally limited to 250–350 pounds. Facilities should apply a sticker to all bariatric equipment with "EC" (for expanded capacity) and a space for the manufacturer's rated weight capacity for that particular equipment model.

■ If patient has partial weight-bearing capability, transfer toward stronger side.

■ Consider using an abdominal binder if the patient's abdomen impairs a patient-handling task.

■ Identify a leader when performing tasks with multiple caregivers. This will assure that the task is synchronized for increased safety of the health care provider and the patient.

■ During any patient transferring task, if any caregiver is required to lift more than 35 pounds of a patient's weight, then the patient should be considered to be fully dependent and assistive devices should be used for the transfer.

FIGURE 4-13 *(continued)*

Bariatric Algorithm 3: Bariatric Reposition in Bed: Side to Side, Up in Bed
rev. 8/23/06

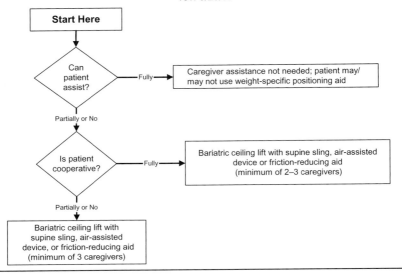

General Notes:
- When pulling a patient up in bed, place the bed flat or in a Trendelenburg position (if tolerated and not medically contraindicated) to aid in gravity; the side rail should be down.
- Avoid shearing force.
- Adjust the height of the bed to elbow height.
- Mobilize the patient as early as possible to avoid weakness resulting from bed rest. This will promote patient independence and reduce the number of high-risk tasks caregivers will provide.
- Consider leaving a friction-reducing device covered with drawsheet under patient at all times to minimize risk to staff during transfers as long as it doesn't negate the pressure-relief qualities of the mattress/overlay.
- Use a sealed, high-density foam wedge to firmly reposition patient on side. Skid-resistant texture materials vary and come in set shapes and cut-your-own rolls. Examples include:
  - Dycem (TM)
  - Scoot-Guard (TM): antimicrobial; clean with soap and water, air dry.
  - Posey-Grip (TM): Posey-Grip does not hold when wet. Washable, reusable, air dry.

- If patient has partial weight-bearing capability, transfer toward stronger side.
- Consider using an abdominal binder if the patient's abdomen impairs a patient-handling task.
- Assure equipment used meets weight requirements. Standard equipment is generally limited to 250–350 pounds. Facilities should apply a sticker to all bariatric equipment with "EC" (for expanded capacity) and a space for the manufacturer's rated weight capacity for that particular equipment model.
- Identify a leader when performing tasks with multiple caregivers. This will assure that the task is synchronized for increased safety of the health care provider and the patient.
- During any patient-handling task, if any caregiver is required to lift more than 35 pounds of a patient's weight, then the patient should be considered to be fully dependent and assistive devices should be used.

FIGURE 4-13 *(continued)*

Bariatric Algorithm 4: Bariatric Reposition in Chair: Wheelchair, Chair, or Dependency Chair
rev. 1/3/06

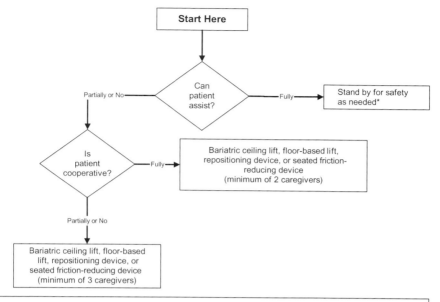

General Notes:
- Take full advantage of chair functions, e.g., chair that reclines, or use an armrest of chair to facilitate repositioning.
- Make sure the chair wheels are locked.
- Consider leaving the sling under the patient at all times to minimize risk to staff during transfers after carefully considering skin risk to patient and the risk of removing/replacing the sling for subsequent moves.

---

*   "Stand by for safety." In most cases, if a bariatric patient is about to fall, there is very little that the caregiver can do to prevent the fall. The caregiver should be prepared to move any items out of the way that could cause injury, try to protect the patient's head from striking any objects or the floor, and seek assistance as needed once the person has fallen.
- If patient has partial weight-bearing capability, transfer toward stronger side.
- Consider using an abdominal binder if the patient's abdomen impairs a patient-handling task.
- Assure equipment used meets weight requirements. Standard equipment is generally limited to 250–350 pounds. Facilities should apply a sticker to all bariatric equipment with "EC" (for expanded capacity) and a space for the manufacturer's rated weight capacity for that particular equipment model.
- Identify a leader when performing tasks with multiple caregivers. This will assure that the task is synchronized for increased safety of the health care provider and the patient.
- During any patient transferring task, if any caregiver is required to lift more than 35 pounds of a patient's weight, then the patient should be considered to be fully dependent and assistive devices should be used for the transfer.

FIGURE 4-13 *(continued)*

**Bariatric Algorithm 5: Patient-Handling Tasks Requiring Access to Body Parts
(Limb, Abdominal Mass, Gluteal Area)**
rev. 1/3/06

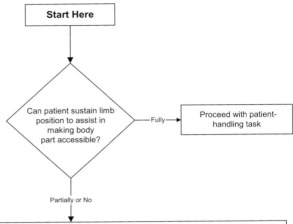

Assemble multidisciplinary team to develop creative solutions that are safe for patient and caregiver.

Examples:

■ Modify use of a full body sling lift to elevate limbs for bathing or wound care (i.e., bariatric limb sling).
■ Use drawsheet with handles for 2 caregivers (1 per side) to elevate abdominal mass to access the perineal area (e.g., catheterization, wound care).
■ To facilitate drying a patient between skin folds, use the air-assisted lateral-transfer aid to blow air or use a hair dryer on a cool setting.
■ Use a sealed, high-density foam wedge to firmly reposition patient on side. Skid-resistant texture materials vary and come in set shapes and cut-your-own rolls. Examples include:
  ■ Dycem (TM)
  ■ Scoot-Guard (TM): antimicrobial; clean with soap and water, air dry.
  ■ Posey-Grip (TM): Posey-Grip does not hold when wet. Washable, reusable, air dry.

■ A multidisciplinary team needs to problem-solve these tasks, communicate to all caregivers, refine as needed, and perform consistently.
■ Consider using an abdominal binder if the patient's abdomen impairs a patient-handling task.
■ During any patient transferring task, if any caregiver is required to lift more than 35 pounds of a patient's weight, then the patient should be considered to be fully dependent and assistive devices should be used for the transfer.

FIGURE 4-13 *(continued)*

Bariatric Algorithm 6: Bariatric Transporting (Stretcher)
rev. 5/1/05

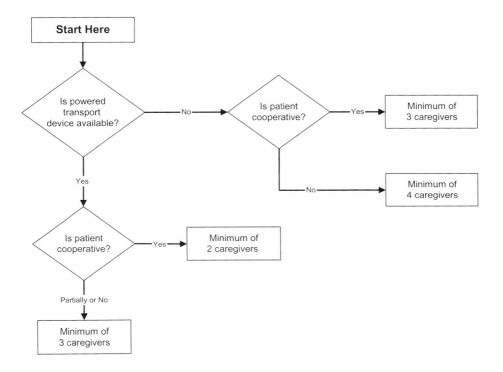

General Notes:
- If the patient has respiratory distress, the stretcher must have the capability of maintaining a high Fowler's position.
- Newer equipment often is easier to propel.
- If patient is uncooperative, secure patient in stretcher.
- During any patient transferring task, if any caregiver is required to lift more than 35 pounds of a patient's weight, then the patient should be considered to be fully dependent and assistive devices should be used for the transfer.

FIGURE 4-13 *(continued)*

Bariatric Algorithm 7: Toileting Tasks for the Bariatric Patient
rev. 8/23/05

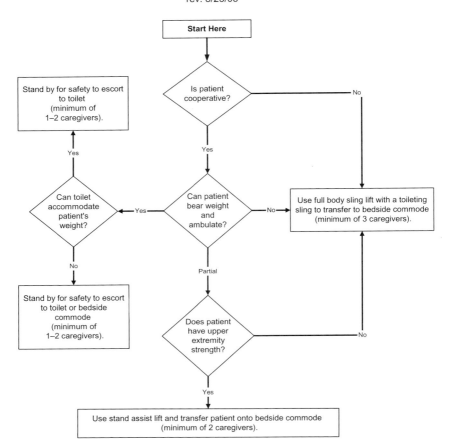

Considerations:
- Is bathroom doorway wide enough to accommodate entry of mechanical lift device and patient?
- Assure equipment used meets weight requirements and is appropriately sized for patient.
- Typically, standard toilets are rated to 350 pounds maximum capacity.
- During any patient transferring task, if any caregiver is required to lift more than 35 pounds of a patient's weight, then the patient should be considered to be fully dependent and assistive devices should be used for the transfer.

FIGURE 4-13 *(continued)*

CHAPTER

5

PREVENTING SLIPS, TRIPS, AND FALLS IN THE HEALTH CARE ENVIRONMENT

THE NATURE OF SLIP, TRIP, AND FALL INJURIES

The terms *slips, trips,* and *falls* have distinctive meanings that become important when identifying causes, assessing risk, and developing controls for prevention. **Slips** result when the foot no longer adequately grips the walking surface. This sudden loss of friction can cause one or both feet to slide freely. With slips, the feet often accelerate forward and the body falls back. The individual may engage in rapid, vigorous movements in an attempt to regain stable footing. Slips do not always result in injury, but injury can occur from a resulting fall or simply from the bodily motion used in the attempt to regain balance. **Trips** are typically caused by the foot catching on something, resulting in a misstep or stumble or a fall. A trip can be caused by as little as a 3/8-inch change in elevation on the walking surface. Typically a trip causes the body to be flung forward. Like slips, trips do not always result in injury, but injury can occur from a resulting fall, or from the bodily motion used in the attempt to regain balance. A **fall** can be defined as the body's downward movement to the floor, ground, or an object. This movement is uncontrolled, unintentional, and sudden. For the purposes of this chapter, falls resulting from being pushed or hit are not included in this definition. Falls often result from slips or trips.

REDUCING FALL RISK IN THE HEALTH CARE ENVIRONMENT

The clinical aspects of client fall prevention are beyond the scope of this chapter. Rather, this chapter will explore some of the common influences and hazards contributing to fall risk in the health care environment. Controlling these influences and hazards can reduce the risk of falls for everyone.

Biomechanical Factors

Biomechanics, simply put, is the study of body motion. As an aspect of ergonomics, biomechanics relates to how an individual moves and walks on surfaces. Thus, ergonomics interventions can impact biomechanics. Individual differences can also impact the way the body moves, whether a client, a caregiver, or a visitor. Individual characteristics serve to emphasize the importance of maintaining a safe care environment for all.

Psychological Factors

Individuals perceive the environment based on their own characteristics. Falls resulting from a **psychological cause** may include those that occur as a result of a lack of awareness of or inability to perceive a hazard. Fall risk can be increased by medical conditions and medication regimens, and by sensory and cognitive impairments such as visual and memory deficits; each of these influences how the environment is viewed.

Caregivers and clients who make an effort to continually scan their environment for hazards are developing a valuable control that may help to reduce risk related to psychological causes. Working efficiently is a work-practice control that can help to avoid unnecessary rushing. Maintaining optimal wellness can also reduce risk related to psychological causes. Additional information on personal wellness can be found in later chapters.

Ergonomics Factors

As discussed in previous chapters, ergonomics involves fitting the work to the worker. It can also refer to fitting the care environment to the client. It includes furnishings, housekeeping, and work- and care-area considerations.

Developing a safe client handling and movement program using client-centered protocols is a critical element to reducing fall hazards. Muscle fatigue may slow reaction time and result in a caregiver misstep or cause the client to become unable to support his or her own weight. This can be a hazard to client and caregiver.

Housekeeping

A clean environment, free of clutter and unnecessary equipment, is an ergonomics control that can reduce the risk of injury. The following work-practice tips can help reduce slip, trip, and fall hazards related to house-keeping:

- Clean up liquids immediately by mopping or using an absorbent material. If the liquid is a chemical, use proper safety procedures (see Chapter 6).

- Sweep up loose debris and discard appropriately.

- Inspect flooring and stair surfaces for holes, chips, or other trip hazards, and follow safety procedures for reporting. Special attention should be given to areas where two different flooring surfaces (such as carpet and vinyl) join.

- Keep stairways clear. Inspect banisters and railings for cleanliness, peeling paint, splintered wood, and other surface abnormalities. Report problems according to facility policy.

- Observe warning signs, safety cones, or barricade tape. If you notice that they are no longer needed, inform the proper personnel.

- Mop only one side of the floor at a time to maintain a dry area of floor surface for walking.

Walking Surfaces

Many falls occur at a **transitional area,** where floor surfaces or surface conditions differ—for example, carpet to smooth flooring, dry to wet flooring—or at areas where the floor surfaces are uneven.

Improving transitions between different flooring surfaces can be accomplished through a combination of engineering and administrative controls. Examples may include leveling raised areas, improving lighting, or adding visual cues such as brightly contrasted floor markings or floor coverings.

Changes in floor maintenance may also be a solution. The floor cleaner used should remove all grease and other slippery residue from the floor. Products are available that clean the floor and leave it with an attractive finish, but do not leave the floor slippery. It may be appropriate to explore such controls in facilities where slip and trip hazards are a particular concern.

Mats may be a suitable solution in some areas. Slip-resistant mats can be used in wet work areas to help maintain good traction. Mats should be made of dense material, should be hard to move, should have a slip-resistant backing to prevent slippage, and should be difficult to fold over on themselves. Special mats may be required for certain areas, such as food-service areas.

Stairways

Stairs should have railings on open sides, and closed stairways should have a railing on at least one side. Railings should be sturdy and firmly affixed. The rails should be kept clean and in good condition. One hand should always be free to grasp the rail. Caregivers and others who must carry items from one floor to another should use the elevator if the load to be carried requires both hands or if the view of the stairs is obstructed. Stairwells and landings should be well lit. It is important that the landing be visually distinct from the stairs, with markings on the edge of each stair. This is typically managed by installing a nonskid tread on the landing and stair edge in contrasting colors.

Walking- and Working-Surface Checklist

OSHA has developed a self-inspection checklist for walking and working surfaces for general industry. Reviewing and using this checklist can assist the caregiver in learning to recognize slip, trip, and fall hazards. Examples from this checklist are provided in Table 5-3.

TABLE 5.3   Walking- and Working-Surface Checklist

General Work Environment:
Is a documented, functioning housekeeping program in place?
Are work surfaces kept dry or are appropriate means taken to ensure the surfaces are slip-resistant?
Are all spilled hazardous materials or liquids, including blood and other potentially infectious materials, cleaned up immediately and according to proper procedures?
Is combustible scrap, debris, and waste stored safely and removed from the work site properly?

Walkways
Are aisles and passageways kept clear?
Are aisles and walkways marked as appropriate?
Are wet surfaces covered with nonslip materials?
Are holes in the floor, sidewalk, or other walking surfaces repaired properly, covered, or otherwise made safe?
Is there safe clearance for walking in aisles where motorized or mechanical handling equipment is operating?
Are materials or equipment stored so that sharp objects will not interfere with the walkway?
Are spilled materials cleaned up immediately?
Are changes of direction or elevation readily identifiable?
Is adequate headroom provided for the entire length of any aisle or walkway?
Are standard guardrails provided wherever aisle or walkway surfaces are elevated more than 30 inches above any adjacent floor or the ground?

Floor and Wall Openings
Are floor openings guarded by a cover, a guardrail, or equivalent on all sides (except at entrances to stairways or ladders)?

(continued)

TABLE 5.3   (continued)

Are grates or similar type covers over floor openings such as floor drains of such design that foot traffic or rolling equipment will not be affected by the grate spacing?

Are floor or wall openings in fire-resistive construction provided with doors or covers compatible with the fire rating of the structure and provided with a self-closing feature when appropriate?

Stairs and Stairways

Are standard stair rails or handrails on all stairways having four or more risers?

Are all stairways at least 22 inches wide?

Do stairs have landing platforms not less than 30 inches in the direction of travel and do they extend 22 inches in width at every 12 feet or less of vertical rise?

Do stairs angle no more than 50 and no less than 30 degrees?

Are step risers on stairs uniform from top to bottom?

Are steps on stairs and stairways designed or provided with a surface that renders them slip-resistant?

Are stairway handrails located between 30 and 34 inches above the leading edge of stair treads?

Do stairway handrails have at least 3 inches of clearance between the handrails and the wall or surface they are mounted on?

Where doors or gates open directly on a stairway, is there a platform provided so the swing of the door does not reduce the width of the platform to less than 21 inches?

Where stairs or stairways exit directly into any area where vehicles may be operated, are adequate barriers and warnings provided to prevent employees stepping into the path of traffic?

Do stairway landings have a dimension measured in the direction of travel, at least equal to the width of the stairway?

Elevated Surfaces

Are signs posted, when appropriate, showing the elevated surface load capacity?

Are surfaces elevated more than 30 inches above the floor or ground provided with standard guardrails?

Is material on elevated surfaces piled, stacked, or racked in a manner to prevent it from tipping, falling, collapsing, rolling, or spreading?

Are dock boards or bridge plates used when transferring materials between docks and trucks or rail cars?

Source: Excerpted from Occupational Safety and Health Administration Self-Inspection Checklists, http://www.osha.gov/SLTC/smallbusiness/chklist.html.

Chairs, Stools, and Ladders

Chairs with spoked bases should have a minimum of five spokes for support. Stools should be available in the work area for overhead reaching tasks. Stools should rest firmly on the floor and have a nonskid tread and a handle that can be used for balance. Using ladders in the workplace requires specialized training. The caregiver should not use a ladder unless this training has been completed. Chairs, beds, tables, or carts should never be used in place of a stool.

Chairs, stools, and ladders should have adequate weight capacity to support the user. This information may be found on the product or in the product literature. If there is any question in this regard, the caregiver should consult with the supervisor.

FOOTWEAR CONSIDERATIONS

Shoes are often not formally considered to be personal protective equipment in health care, but shoe selection is important to foot health and safety. Some individuals have special footwear needs. Although similar considerations for foot safety and health apply, individuals with foot health concerns should see their physician for advice on proper footwear.

Choosing a Good Shoe

When choosing shoes to help prevent slips, trips, and falls, it is important to select a shoe that is slip- and oil-resistant. The caregiver should assess the shoe **outsole,** or the bottom of the shoe, to determine slip resistance. The outsole also provides shock-absorptive qualities to the shoe. For optimal slip resistance, the outsole should have a raised tread pattern that extends over the entire bottom of the shoe. Shoes with soles that "curl" up in the front, typical of some running shoes, can catch on certain types of flooring and create a trip hazard. Generally, a softer outsole provides better traction indoors. The outsole should be flat and should have flexible construction. The caregiver should consider a low (less than 1 inch) wedged outsole for indoor occupational footwear, with a closed toe and heel.

The part of the shoe that encloses the foot, or the **upper,** should be made of a soft material that gives, yet offers moisture resistance. Care should be taken to avoid shoes with seams in high-pressure areas, especially trouble spots like bunions. Lace-up shoes tend to provide better support to the foot, and more easily accommodate insoles and other devices that may be needed for foot health. The shoe should provide a deep heel cup to protect and support the protective tissues of the heel. The heel cup should fit snugly and cushion the heel, with minimal slippage. The back of the shoe should be closed. An open-heeled shoe can easily slip off, and may throw the wearer off balance and result in an ankle injury or a fall. This is an important consideration when recommending client slipper selection to the family, and for caregiver footwear. Open-backed slippers and shoes are common, but may not be the best choice for the health care environment. The natural spread of the toes is important to balance, so providing a roomy toe box that fits the shape of the foot and allows the toes to spread naturally may reduce fall risk. A closed toe adds a measure of hygiene protection against unintentional spills and a measure of safety protection against injury resulting from striking the foot.

Comfort

Shoes should be comfortable when they are tried on for the first time. It is a good idea to have both feet measured each time shoes are purchased and to shop for shoes at the end of the day, when the feet are slightly larger. The shoe style should conform as closely as possible to the shape of the foot. The caregiver should stand and walk during the fitting process to ensure that there is adequate space for the great toe at the end of the shoe and to check that the ball of the foot fits snugly into the widest part of the shoe.

Monitoring Work Shoes

Just like any piece of equipment, shoes need to be maintained and monitored for wear and tear. The shoes should be kept clean and inspected regularly for damage. Regardless of tread, shoes should be replaced when they are no longer comfortable.

Wear Patterns as Clues

Bulging or excessive wear over the lateral or medial side of the shoe upper, wear-through in the toe box, a cracking sound when grasping the back part of the upper near the heel, or excessive wear or tearing of the lining of the upper may signal a need to replace footwear. Shoes should be replaced when they become worn. Some wear patterns can be indicative of a shoe/foot mismatch or potentially troublesome foot-related health conditions. The caregiver should seek the assistance of a professional specializing in foot health, such as a podiatrist, if there is a concern.

USING THE HIERARCHY OF CONTROLS TO REDUCE FALL RISK RELATED TO ENVIRONMENTAL HAZARDS

Hazard elimination and engineering controls are typically the best long-term solution for correcting slip, trip, and fall hazards in the care environment, but may take time to implement.

Work-practice and administrative controls are used extensively in preventing falls. Posters, warning signs, and training are examples. Policies and procedures are also examples. Reporting falls and near misses is an important control, and most facilities have a reporting policy in place.

PART 2

CHEMICAL SAFETY AND AIRBORNE EXPOSURES

CHAPTER

6

WORKING SAFELY WITH DRUGS AND OTHER SUBSTANCES

INTRODUCTION

*C*hemicals *are composed of unique configurations of atoms, ions, or groups of atoms. In the broadest sense of the word, all substances are chemicals or chemical mixtures. We don't need to be concerned with every chemical, only with those that may cause harm. Chemical hazards were described briefly in earlier chapters as those chemicals with potential to cause harm, or adverse* health effects, *if unprotected exposure occurs. A health effect is simply a change to the body that may occur in response to a chemical exposure. Health effects may be beneficial, as with a medication, or harmful, such as an illness linked to a hazardous chemical exposure. This chapter will discuss hazardous chemicals in more depth.*

WHAT IS A HAZARDOUS CHEMICAL?

Unprotected exposure to hazardous chemicals in the workplace is a serious problem. A **cancer** is a growth caused when cells multiply uncontrollably and healthy tissue is destroyed. Chemicals and other substances known to cause cancer are called **carcinogens.** Formaldehyde is an example of a carcinogen. **Asthma** is a respiratory condition, typically triggered by allergies, resulting in constricted airways. Symptoms include coughing and difficulty breathing. Chemicals that may lead to allergic reactions in susceptible individuals are called **sensitizers.** Latex is an example of a sensitizer of special concern to caregivers.

Chemicals that damage the **hematopoietic system** erode the body's ability to make blood cells. Other chemicals may interfere with the oxygen-carrying capacity of the blood (carbon monoxide, for example), or prevent the body from using oxygen properly, such as cyanide. **Irritants** are chemicals that can cause irritation of the skin in susceptible individuals. **Hepatotoxins, nephrotoxins,** and **neurotoxins** are chemicals that can harm the liver, kidneys, and nervous system, respectively. These are called **target organ chemicals.** A target organ (including the skin or eyes) is an organ that may be affected by toxic properties of a hazardous chemical in susceptible individuals. Some hazardous chemicals have more than one target organ.

OSHA's Hazard Communication Standard

The Hazard Communication (HazCom) Standard was written by OSHA to ensure that the hazards of all chemicals produced or imported are evaluated and that information concerning their hazards is transmitted to employers and employees. OSHA directed that the information would be provided by using comprehensive hazard communication programs, developed by each employer, that include container labeling and other forms of warning, employee training, and material safety data sheets (MSDSs). The MSDS is intended to convey information about the characteristics, hazards, and controls for hazardous chemicals or chemical mixtures used in the workplace.

The HazCom Standard, 29 Code of Federal Regulations Part 1910.1200, defines a hazardous chemical as "any chemical which is a physical hazard or a health hazard." Physical hazards include chemicals with scientific evidence to support that they have properties that can cause sudden injury. This category includes explosives or chemicals that form explosive atmospheres, as well as combustible liquids, flammables, compressed gases, reactive chemicals, organic peroxides, oxidizers, or **pyrophorics** (chemicals that spontaneously ignite in air). A **health hazard** is an agent or chemical substance for which there is there is scientific evidence to show that exposure may cause adverse health outcomes in susceptible employees who may be exposed. Health hazards may have an acute effect but may also do damage over time, resulting in a chronic health condition. OSHA defines health hazards as chemicals that are carcinogens, toxic or highly toxic agents, reproductive toxins, irritants, corrosives, sensitizers, hepatotoxins, nephrotoxins, neurotoxins, agents that act on the hematopoietic system, and agents that damage the lungs, skin, eyes, or mucous membranes.

CHEMICALS IN HEALTH CARE—WHAT MAKES THEM DISTINCTIVE?

The common thread with all drugs and many chemicals used in health care is biological activity. Whether the target is bacteria, a virus, a cancer cell, or another human cell, all drugs and many chemicals are used because they cause a specific biological reaction. Whenever a chemical or drug affects a cell in one way, the possibility exists that it can affect people in other ways as well. For example, benzalkonium chloride is a quaternary ammonia preparation commonly used in disinfectants. It is also a suspected **asthmagen** (a chemical that may cause asthma). Many antineoplastic drugs, or cancer drugs, as they are sometimes called, are carcinogens. Even some antibiotics have shown evidence of being hazardous to the caregiver administering the medication.

Drugs

Because of their biological activity, almost all drugs meet the OSHA definition of a hazardous chemical; however, the HazCom Standard treats drugs somewhat differently from other hazardous chemicals, mostly because they are already regulated by other federal agencies. For example, drugs are exempt from the labeling requirements under the HazCom Standard. Certain drugs are exempt from the standard altogether. These drugs include any drug—as that term is defined in the Federal Food, Drug, and Cosmetic Act—when it is in solid, final form for direct administration to the client (e.g., tablets or pills); drugs that are packaged by the chemical manufacturer for sale to consumers in a retail establishment (e.g., over-the-counter drugs); and drugs intended for personal consumption by employees while in the workplace (e.g., first-aid supplies).

Injectables and other drugs that must be mixed, or otherwise do not meet the above definition, are covered by the HazCom Standard, and the employer is required to comply with all elements of the HazCom Standard (except labeling). (See Figure 6-1.) This includes informing the caregiver about the hazards associated with administering the drug, as well as providing the necessary controls needed for the caregiver to work with the drug safely. Controls may include a ventilation hood, gloves, a respirator, or other control specific to that drug.

MATERIAL SAFETY DATA SHEETS

A MSDS is a document that contains information about the characteristics and hazards of a particular hazardous chemical or chemical mixture. The MSDS is produced by the chemical manufacturer or

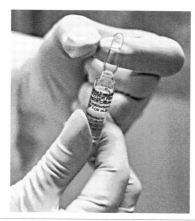

FIGURE 6-1 *Drugs are generally considered hazardous chemicals. Except for drugs packaged for retail sale, for personal use, and tablets and pills in final form for direct administration to the client, all drugs are covered by the Hazard Communication Standard. Because drugs are highly regulated by other agencies, they are exempt from the labeling requirement, but all other provisions of the Hazard Communication Standard apply, including having a current material safety data sheet.*

importer and must be in English (at a minimum). Each MSDS is required to convey specific information about the chemical or chemical mixture, including the appropriate controls needed to work safely. Employers are required to have an MSDS in the workplace for each hazardous chemical used and are required to train employees on how to use the information on the MSDS.

Understanding MSDSs

The MSDS is often dismissed as an inconvenient OSHA requirement, but the information on the MSDS can be used in many ways to improve workplace safety. For example, the information on the MSDS includes hazardous properties of the chemical, the potential **routes of exposure** (ways the chemical can enter the body), the methods used to control exposure to the chemical, and the appropriate response should an exposure or spill occur. A **spill** is simply an unintentional leak, or discharge, of the chemical from its container. Caregivers who take the time to read and understand the MSDSs for chemicals they work with are much better prepared to use the chemical safely—without suffering a health effect.

Although OSHA does not mandate the format or order of presentation of the hazard information, the agency does require that certain information be provided. A sample MSDS can be found in Figure 6-2.

MATERIAL SAFETY DATA SHEET

I – PRODUCT IDENTIFICATION

COMPANY NAME: We Wash Inc.

Tel No: (314) 621-1818

ADDRESS: 5035 Manchester Avenue

Nights: (314) 621-1399

Freedom, Texas 79430

CHEMTREC: (800) 424-9343

PRODUCT NAME: Spotfree

Product No.: 2190

Synonyms: Warewashing Detergent

II – HAZARDOUS INGREDIENTS OF MIXTURES

MATERIAL:	(CAS#)	% By Wt.	TLV	PEL

According to the OSHA Hazard Communication Standard,

29CFR 1910.1200,   N/A   N/A   N/A

this product contains no hazardous ingredients.

III – PHYSICAL DATA

Vapor Pressure, mm Hg: N/A

Vapor Density (Air = 1) 60–90F: N/A

Evaporation Rate (ether = 1): N/A

% Volatile by wt N/A

Solubility in H_2O: Complete

pH @ 1%   Solution 9.3–9.8

Freezing Point F: N/A

pH as Distributed: N/A

Boiling Point F: N/A

Appearance: Off-White granular powder

Specific Gravity H_2O = 1 @25C: N/A

Odor: Mild Chemical Odor

IV – FIRE AND EXPLOSION

Flash Point F: N/AV

Flammable Limits: N/A

Extinguishing Media: The product is not flammable or combustible. Use media appropriate for the primary source of fire. Special Firefighting Procedures: Use caution when fighting any fire involving chemicals. A self-contained breathing apparatus is essential.

Unusual Fire and Explosion Hazards: None Known

V – REACTIVITY DATA

Solubility–Conditions to avoid: None Known

Compatibility: Contact of carbonates or bicarbonates with acids can release large quantities of carbon dioxide and heat.

Hazardous Decomposition Products: In fire situations heat decomposition may result in the release of sulfur oxides.

Conditions Contributing to Hazardous Polymerization: N/A

FIGURE 6-2 Sample material safety data sheet (MSDS). *The MSDS contains information about chemical properties of the product, including, but not limited to, possible health effects and protective measures that can be taken to prevent them.*

Spotfree
VI – HEALTH HAZARD DATA

EFFECTS OF OVEREXPOSURE (Medical Conditions Aggravated/Target Organ Effects)
A. ACUTE (Primary Route of Exposure) EYES: Product granules may cause mechanical irritation to eyes. SKIN (Primary Route of Exposure): Prolonged repeated contact with skin may result in drying on skin. INGESTION: Not expected to be toxic if swallowed, however, gastrointestinal discomfort may occur.
B. SUBCHRONIC, CHRONIC, OTHER: None known.

VII – EMERGENCY AND FIRST-AID PROCEDURES

EYES: In case of contact, flush thoroughly with water for 15 minutes. Get medical attention if irritation persists.
SKIN: Flush any dry Spotfree from skin with flowing water. Always wash hands after use.
INGESTION: If swallowed, drink large quantities of water and call a physician.

VIII – SPILL OR LEAK PROCEDURES

Spill Management: Sweep up material and repackage if possible.
   Spill residue may be flushed to the sewer with water.

Waste Disposal Methods: Dispose of in accordance with federal, state, and local regulations.

IX – PROTECTION INFORMATION/CONTROL MEASURES

Respiratory: None needed

Eye: Safety glasses

Glove: Not required

Other Clothing and Equipment: None required

Ventilation: Normal

X – SPECIAL PRECAUTIONS

Precautions to be taken in Handling and Storing: Avoid contact with eyes. Avoid prolonged or repeated contact with skin. Wash thoroughly after handling. Keep container closed when not in use.

Additional Information: Store away from acids.

Prepared by: D. Martinez

Revision Date: 04/11/XX

Seller makes no warranty, expressed or implied, concerning the use of this product other than indicated on the label. Buyer assumes all risk of use and/or handling of this material when such use and/or handling is contrary to label instructions.

While Seller believes that the information contained herein is accurate, such information is offered solely for its customers' consideration and verification under their specific use conditions. This information is not to be deemed a warranty or representation of any kind for which Seller assumes legal responsibility.

FIGURE 6-2 *(continued)*

Key Elements of the MSDS

MSDSs can contain a great deal of information, much of it targeted toward specific groups. Some MSDSs are more complete than others; sometimes the information provided may be too general. The caregiver should take the initiative to bring concerns to the supervisor, who may call the manufacturer to get more specific information.

Manufacturer Contact Information

The manufacturer contact information is on the MSDS for when something nonroutine occurs, such as an exposure or spill.

Hazardous Components

Preparers of MSDSs are required to include the exact chemical name as well as common trade names. With few exceptions, hazardous chemicals that make up more than 1% of the ingredients (0.1% for carcinogens) in a product must be listed in this section.

Exposure Limits

"Acceptable" exposure levels can typically be found in the exposure limits section of the MSDS. Often, there will be two limits listed on the MSDS, a **threshold limit value (TLV)** and a **permissible exposure limit (PEL)**. It is important to understand the difference between these.

The TLV is an exposure limit guideline developed by the American Conference of Governmental Industrial Hygienists (ACGIH) and is based on scientific study. It reflects the level of exposure that an average worker can experience without unreasonable risk of adverse health effects, without regard to the economic and technical feasibility of controls. The ACGIH updates the listing regularly as new health-risk evidence emerges. The TLVs are guidelines and are not enforceable.

In contrast, the PEL is essentially the maximum amount of an airborne chemical to which a worker can be exposed under OSHA regulations. The most familiar PEL relates to an employee's average airborne exposure in any 8-hour work shift over a 40-hour workweek. Additional PELs have been established for other types of exposures that require more stringent limits. The PELs have not been updated since their inception in 1968. These levels are more than guidelines; they are legally enforceable.

Over time, OSHA began to identify chemicals that presented special health risks. Expanded health standards were developed to address these hazards. These standards typically address a specific chemical and, along with PELs, require additional employer actions to control the hazard.

Reactivity Data

The section on reactivity data provides information on product stability and incompatibility. All too often, MSDSs do not list what specific chemicals may be incompatible. Specific incompatibility is important information to have, because such chemical reactions can be violent or create a more serious health hazard. The caregiver should take the initiative to bring concerns to the supervisor, who may call the manufacturer to get more specific information.

Health Effects

The MSDS may include the health hazard category (e.g., irritant, sensitizer, etc.), the specific health effect (e.g., dermatitis, asthma), or both for a specific chemical or drug. Target organs may also be specified. This section is especially valuable to the caregiver who has a symptom, and wonders if it may be linked to an exposure.

The health effects of exposure to hazardous chemicals and drugs can be varied. The risk of health-hazard exposure relates to toxicity, dose, and individual differences. Toxicity relates to the chemical potency, or ability to produce an adverse health effect. Dose considers the duration and frequency of exposure, as well as the quantity of chemical involved. In a chemical exposure, dose can be evaluated through environmental monitoring to measure the level of contaminant in the air (how much) as compared to the published TLVs and PELs previously discussed. These levels are typically averaged over an 8-hour day. The industrial hygienist then evaluates the frequency of the task involving the chemical (how often) and how long the task takes (how long, or duration). If the exposure is too high, additional controls may be needed. If they are low, no action is required. It is important to note that air monitoring cannot measure the actual dose received by an individual; it can only quantify the exposure. Because all humans are different, some individuals can be exposed to safe levels, at or below the exposure limit, with no ill effects, while others become ill. When the employer has met the legal requirements to control a specific hazard and the caregiver still suffers, it may be in the caregiver's best interest to seek alternative employment opportunities.

Routes of Exposure

It is important for caregivers to be familiar with the routes of exposure for chemicals they use. Exposure routes include inhalation, skin absorption, skin contact, ingestion, and injection. Inhalation and skin absorption are the most common routes of chemical exposure in health care. Chemical exposure through **inhalation** can result from breathing in air containing chemical vapors, fumes, or gases. Exposure to chemicals through inhalation can cause local effects in the respiratory system, as well as systemic effects as a result of the chemical traveling throughout the circulatory system of the body to the various organs and tissues. **Skin absorption** is the process of a chemical or drug being drawn into the body through the pores of the skin or through the mucous membranes, especially around the eyes. Health effects from skin absorption in susceptible individuals can also be either local or systemic. **Skin contact** is a route of exposure whereby a chemical or drug acts locally on the skin surface, with health effects generally limited to the exposure site, but some skin contact hazards may also damage skin integrity, allowing skin absorption. The **ingestion** route of exposure is oral consumption by eating or drinking. Many medications are delivered intentionally through the ingestion route. Chemical hazard exposure may occur by consuming food or beverages contaminated with the chemical, or as a result of poor hand hygiene. In health care, exposure through **injection** can result anytime the skin is punctured by a contaminated sharp object; it is not necessarily limited to injectable medications or needle sticks.

Emergency and First-Aid Procedures

The MSDS provides basic first-aid measures to be initiated in the event of an unprotected exposure or overexposure. It is imperative that a process be established whereby the MSDS is supplied to the provider anytime an employee presents for medical care as a result of an exposure.

Safe Handling

Each MSDS provides basic information for the handling, storage, and disposal of the chemical. The information may include storage incompatibilities, temperature ranges for storage, appropriate spill response measures, and special waste disposal considerations.

Control Measures

The control measures section of MSDSs contains information on controls necessary to use the chemical safely, with information on ventilation, respiratory protection, eye protection, and protective clothing, including glove selection. As noted earlier, however, not all manufacturers provide the necessary information on the MSDS. Other sources of information may need to be consulted.

Ventilation is an engineering control. It is often mentioned in the controls section of the MSDS either as general ventilation or local exhaust ventilation. **General ventilation** is ventilation encountered in most office buildings and health care facilities. Fresh air enters the ventilation system and is filtered and mixed with recycled air from the building environment and delivered to the occupants. General ventilation is adequate for most low-hazard chemicals. **Local exhaust ventilation** is typically used for disagreeable odors and more toxic chemicals. The contaminant is captured by a special air handling system and removed from the area. The air may be filtered and recycled to the general ventilation or filtered and exhausted out of doors.

Spill Response

This section of the MSDS is most likely to contain sketchy information, such as "follow local and state regulations." Spill response is covered by the OSHA Hazardous Waste Operations and Emergency Response (**HAZWOPER**) Standard, which specifies the employer requirements when addressing spills of hazardous chemicals. There are two basic options available to employers when dealing with spill response. The company can designate, train, and equip employees to respond and clean the spill, or the employer can rely on an outside emergency response team, typically the local fire department hazardous materials unit.

One of the more difficult issues in spill response is identifying an incidental spill from an emergency spill. An **incidental spill** is an unintentional discharge or leak of hazardous chemical that does not present a significant risk to employees in the immediate vicinity or to those cleaning it up. Generally, incidental spills are those that may be safely cleaned up by employees who are knowledgeable about the chemical and its controls. In contrast, an **emergency spill** is an unintentional discharge or leak of chemical hazard that may lead to a situation that is immediately dangerous to life or health. Generally, incidental spills are not emergencies. The challenge is in determining how much of a particular chemical, if spilled, could create toxic exposure levels or dangerous situations. The employer should do this evaluation for each chemical and communicate the results to the employees who use the hazardous chemical.

Labeling

The HazCom Standard requires that all chemicals be labeled with the identity of the hazardous chemicals in the mixture, appropriate hazard warnings, including which organ or system is affected, and contact information for the manufacturer (or responsible party). Hazardous chemicals that are transferred to secondary smaller containers must also be labeled with this information unless the chemical is for immediate use (during the same work shift) by the caregiver who performed the transfer. Other labeling systems, such as numerical rating systems, can be used if the caregiver has been trained on how to interpret them. Look at the examples of numerical labeling systems in Figures 6-5 and 6-6.

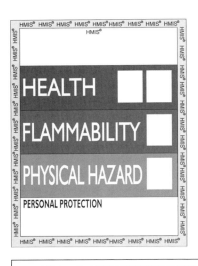

Explanation of the HMIS® Ratings

HMIS® III - HEALTH HAZARD RATINGS

* Chronic Hazard Chronic (long-term) health effects may result from repeated overexposure
0 Minimal Hazard No significant risk to health
1 Slight Hazard Irritation or minor reversible injury possible
2 Moderate Hazard Temporary or minor injury may occur
3 Serious Hazard Major injury likely unless prompt action is taken and medical treatment is given
4 Severe Hazard Life-threatening, major or permanent damage may result from single or repeated overexposures

HMIS® III - FLAMMABILITY RATINGS

0 Minimal Hazard Materials that will not burn
1 Slight Hazard Materials that must be preheated before ignition will occur. Includes liquids, solids and semisolids having a flash point above 200° F. (Class IIIB)
2 Moderate Hazard Materials which must be moderately heated or exposed to high ambient temperatures before ignition will occur. Includes liquids having a flash point at or above 100° F but below 200° F. (Classes II & IIIA)
3 Serious Hazard Materials capable of ignition under almost all normal temperature conditions. Includes flammable liquids with flash points below 73° F and boiling points above 100° F, as well as liquids with flash points between 73° F and 100° F. (Classes IB & IC)
4 Severe Hazard Flammable gases, or very volatile flammable liquids with flash points below 73° F, and boiling points below 100° F. Materials may ignite spontaneously with air. (Class IA)

HMIS® III - PHYSICAL HAZARD RATINGS

0 Minimal Hazard Materials that are normally stable, even under fire conditions, and will NOT react with water, polymerize, decompose, condense, or self-react. Non-explosives.
1 Slight Hazard Materials that are normally stable but can become unstable (self-react) at high temperatures and pressures. Materials may react non-violently with water or undergo hazardous polymerization in the absence of inhibitors.
2 Moderate Hazard Materials that are unstable and may undergo violent chemical changes at normal temperature and pressure with low risk for explosion. Materials may react violently with water or form peroxides upon exposure to air.
3 Serious Hazard Materials that may form explosive mixtures with water and are capable of detonation or explosive reaction in the presence of a strong initiating source. Materials may polymerize, decompose, self-react, or undergo other chemical change at normal temperature and pressure with moderate risk of explosion.
4 Severe Hazard Materials that are readily capable of explosive water reaction, detonation or explosive decomposition, polymerization, or self-reaction at normal temperature and pressure.

FIGURE 6-5 Hazardous Materials Information System (HMIS®) labeling system.
The health hazard section is blue, the flammability section is red, and the physical hazard section is orange. (Courtesy of National Paint and Coatings Association. HMIS® is a registered trademark and service mark of the National Paintings and Coatings Association [NPCA] NPCA has exclusively licensed J.J. Keller & Associates, Inc. to print and distribute HMIS® labels and related materials.)

BLUE: HEATH HAZARD
4 = Danger: May be fatal
3 = Warning: Corrosive or toxic
2 = Warning: Harmful if inhaled
1 = Caution: May cause irritation
0 = No unusual hazard

YELLOW REACTIVITY
4 = Danger: Explosive at room temperature
3 = Danger: May be explosive if spark occurs or if heated under confinement
2 = Warning: Unstable or may react if mixed with water
1 = Caution: May react if heated or mixed with water
0 = Stable: Nonreactive when mixed with water

RED: FIRE HAZARD
4 = Danger: Flammable gas or extremely flammable liquid
3 = Warning: Flammable liquid
2 = Caution: Combustible liquid
1 = Caution: Combustible if heated
0 = Noncombustible

WHITE: PPE
A Goggles
B Goggles, gloves
C Goggles, gloves, apron
D Face shields, gloves, apron
E Goggles, gloves, mask
F Goggles, gloves, apron, mask
X Gloves

(a)

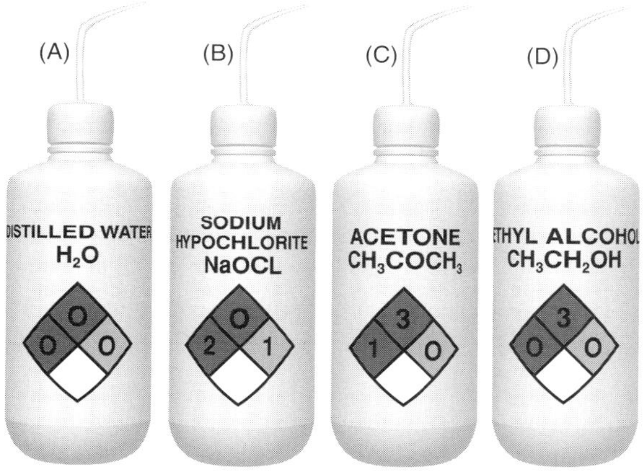

(b)

FIGURE 6-6 National Fire Protection Association (NFPA) labeling system. *The NFPA labeling system is widely used, especially in laboratories:*
(a) The colors and respective hazard categories in the NFPA labeling system. Notice that the color coding for the hazard categories in this NFPA system is consistent with color coding of the HMIS® system illustrated in Figure 6-5.
(b) Four containers are marked using the NFPA color and number method for identifying and warning of chemical hazards: (A) distilled water: presents no health, fire, or reactivity hazard and requires no personal protective equipment when used (all areas represented by zeros); (B) sodium hypochlorite: does not promote a fire hazard (red/0), is harmful if inhaled (blue/2), and may react if heated or mixed with water (yellow/1); (C) acetone: a flammable liquid (red/3), may cause irritation (blue/1), stable and nonreactive when mixed with water (yellow/0); (D) ethyl alcohol: a flammable liquid (red/3), no unusual health hazard (blue/0), and stable and nonreactive when mixed with water (yellow/0). (Courtesy of POL Consultants, 2 Russ Farm Way, Delanco, NJ 08075, 856-824-0800)

Training and Informing Employees

All employees who use or who may be exposed to hazardous chemicals must be provided with information and training at the time of their initial assignment and whenever a new hazardous chemical is introduced into the work area. The information and training may be chemical specific or it may address hazard categories (for example, irritants or flammables).

The information provided to employees must include the requirements of the HazCom Standard, any activities in the work areas where hazardous chemicals are present, and the locations of the HazCom Program, chemical inventory, and MSDSs.

Training must address ways an employee can identify the release or presence of a hazardous chemical, the physical and health hazards associated with the chemicals in use, the controls to be used, and the details of the written HazCom Program. The employer is required to provide an explanation of the labeling system and the MSDS, as well as how employees can access and use hazard information.

TRADE SECRETS

Bona fide trade secrets are exempt from certain requirements of the HazCom Standard under certain circumstances. For example, the specific chemical identity (including the chemical name) may be withheld from the MSDS as long as the hazards are disclosed to the treating provider in a medical emergency or are disclosed to provide medical or other occupational health services to employees in nonemergent circumstances. The manufacturer may require the request to be in writing and require a signed confidentiality agreement. In exposure situations involving trade secrets, it is especially important to provide the treating physician with a copy of the MSDS so the manufacturer can be contacted promptly.

CHAPTER

7

INDOOR AIR QUALITY IN HEALTH CARE—GOOD AIR FOR GOOD HEALTH

INTRODUCTION

The art of managing risks involves using tools and techniques to assess and minimize the chances for adverse consequences. Indoor air quality is a risk that can be managed. **Indoor air quality (IAQ)** *refers to the nature, or characteristics, of indoor air that may affect the health and well-being of occupants. Although this definition applies broadly to all constructed environments, IAQ generally refers to nonmanufacturing work environments such as office buildings, hospitals, and schools, and similar work settings.*

AMBIENT AIR QUALITY

Ambient air quality can be defined as the condition of the air in the surrounding environment. Poor ambient air quality has been associated with an increased incidence of respiratory ailments, particularly in populations with existing respiratory conditions. The use of coal for hundreds of years has led to an escalation in airborne **pollutant emissions,** which are substances that harm the environment when mixed with soil, water, or air.

There is a growing body of scientific evidence indicating that indoor air can, in some situations, be more polluted than outdoor air. Contributing factors include construction of "tighter" buildings, reducing fresh air intake in the interest of energy conservation, lack of building maintenance, increased use of synthetic building materials and furnishings, and occupant-generated contaminants, such as body odor and fragrances.

INDOOR AIR QUALITY

Indoor air quality encompasses contaminants that potentially pollute indoor air, as well as the nonhazardous qualities of air such as temperature, humidity, nuisance odors, and carbon dioxide buildup that can subjectively affect building occupant comfort and well-being.

Indoor Air Quality Problems

Indoor air quality problems can be caused by ventilation system deficiencies; building occupants themselves; indoor sources that release gases, vapors, or particles; or a combination of these. Building occupants can contribute to poor IAQ by improper hygiene practices, using fragrances, blocking air vents, improper watering and maintenance of office plants, or infrequent or improper disposal of garbage. Less than ideal temperature and humidity conditions, poor lighting, and nuisance or hazardous noise levels can also present challenges. Other contributing factors include ergonomics and psychosocial hazards and risk factors.

For indoor air to pose an injury or illness risk, there must be a source of contamination, a pathway of exposure (such as through a ventilation system or an open door), and a route of exposure, such as inhalation, ingestion, or skin or mucous membrane absorption. This concept is illustrated in Figure 7-1.

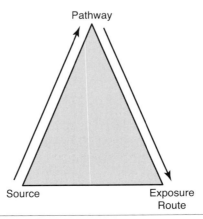

Pathway

Source

Exposure
Route

FIGURE 7-1 Exposure paradigm.

Focusing on potential sources of indoor air pollution can sometimes help lead to a diagnosis of, and remedy for, an IAQ problem. In other cases, in spite of rigorous investigation, a source is never found.

Sick Building Syndrome

Sick building syndrome (SBS) is a specific term used to describe cases in which 20% or more building occupants report adverse acute health and comfort effects that appear to be linked to the time they spend in the building, but in which no specific illness can be identified. Many different symptoms have been associated with SBS; including headache; respiratory problems; irritation of the eyes, nose, and throat; fatigue; reduced concentration; and irritability. The concerns involved with SBS tend to be nonspecific and nonclinically observable.

Building-Related Illness

Building-related illness (BRI) refers to an illness brought on by exposure to the building air, in which symptoms of diagnosable illness are identified and can be *directly* attributed to specific agents in the air. Examples of building-related illnesses with symptoms, potential causes, and prevalence are provided in Table 7-1.

TABLE 7-1   Potential Building-Related Illnesses, Symptoms, Potential Causes, and Prevalence

BRI	Symptoms	Potential Causes	Prevalence
Carbon monoxide poisoning	Headache, dizziness, discoloration, positive blood test, coma	Uncontrolled combustion, elevated carbon monoxide concentrations	Rare
Aspergillosis	Fever, malaise, cough, coughing up blood or brownish mucous plugs, weight loss	Aspergillus species and weakened immune system	Rare
Irritation	Watering, burning, or dryness of the eyes, nose, and throat	Excessive concentrations of volatile organic chemicals such as solvents or formaldehyde; exacerbated by very dry air	Moderate
Legionnaire's disease/ Pontiac fever	Muscle aches, stiffness, joint pain, loss of energy, malaise, headache, fever, chills, nonproductive cough, difficulty breathing, chest pain	Inhalation of Legionella bacteria from warm, moist, water systems, including ventilation systems	Rare

Source: www.epa.gov.

The Importance of Ventilation

Indoor air quality problems are often related to the heating, ventilation, and air-conditioning system. As a result, troubleshooting resources are often concentrated in this area in an effort to resolve indoor air quality problems.

As depicted in Figure 7-1, in addition to considering the source, it is also important to focus on the pollutant pathway. Outdoor air enters and leaves a building by infiltration, natural ventilation, and mechanical ventilation. **Infiltration** refers to the gradual flow of air into a building through openings, joints, and cracks in walls, floors and ceilings, and around windows and doors. In natural ventilation, air moves through opened windows and doors. Air movement by both infiltration and natural ventilation is caused by temperature differences between indoors and outdoors in addition to wind.

Mechanical ventilation devices vary, but in health care they are commonly complex air-handling systems called **heating, ventilation, and air-conditioning (HVAC) systems** that use fans, filtration, and ductwork to continuously remove indoor air and distribute filtered and conditioned outdoor air throughout a facility.

The outdoor air entering the system must come from an outdoor air intake. The location of this intake is critical to prevent re-entrainment of other outdoor pollution sources. **Re-entrainment** is a situation that occurs when the air being exhausted from a building is immediately brought back into the system through the air intake and other openings in the building and redistributed.

The design, care, and maintenance of the ventilation system are important in preventing IAQ problems and managing buildings for optimal quality indoor air.

Key Elements of a Successful IAQ Program

A successful IAQ program bears the same components of other successful health and safety programs. In addition, an IAQ program should include:

- Visible management commitment in support of the IAQ program and to provide an environment with quality indoor air.

- Achievable goals for the IAQ program, and a method for measuring success.

- A culture that welcomes ideas to improve IAQ in the work setting.

- A verbalized expectation that good IAQ is everyone's responsibility.

- Provisions for accurate information about factors contributing to IAQ.

- Clear responsibilities for IAQ management.

- Follow-up and documentation of IAQ concerns.

Preventive Maintenance Programs

HVAC preventive maintenance programs emerge as perhaps the most powerful prevention tool in managing indoor air quality. Although the caregiver will not be involved in this aspect of IAQ, it is important to know that it is happening. Most facility support personnel have a thorough understanding of the overall system design and its intended function and limitations.

Walk-through Inspections and Testing

The walk-through is a tour of the facility with the intent of getting a good overview of ongoing activities and building functions and to look for potential IAQ problems. The industrial hygienist is often asked to anticipate potential exposures, provide technical assistance to personnel involved with IAQ, and, in some instances, conduct sampling to determine airflow patterns, ventilation adequacy, or airborne concentrations of specific indoor contaminants.

Clear Communication

With clear and open communication as a part of the IAQ process, many problems can be prevented. When problems do arise, they can be more easily and promptly remedied.

IAQ CHALLENGES

As previously mentioned, although most IAQ problems can be easily remedied, there are cases in which rigorous investigation does not reveal a cause for an indoor air quality problem. Some of these cases may be related to transient outdoor contaminants that made their way into the building for a brief period, for example, from a passing train. In other cases, common building contaminants may be present at the very low levels typical in most buildings, but an individual is having symptoms. These levels are not bothersome to most individuals, but, as with other chemicals, a few individuals may, because of their unique characteristics and physical condition, experience symptoms as a result of these low-level exposures. Unfortunately, there is little that can be done for these individuals. Industrial hygiene sampling is generally of limited value in these cases. There are no threshold limit values (TLVs) or permissible exposure limit (PELs) for the nonindustrial environment, so, except for radon, there are few standard benchmarks with which to compare, even if sampling is performed.

PART 3

DISEASE PREVENTION

CHAPTER

8

DISEASE TRANSMISSION BASICS

INTRODUCTION

*D*iseases capable of being transmitted and causing infection are called **communicable diseases**. These diseases are caused by pathogens. A **pathogen** is a microorganism, usually a fungus, bacteria, virus, or parasite, capable of causing disease. The capacity of a pathogen to cause disease relates to its capability to grow and reproduce (**virulence**) and its ability to invade tissue. A description of specific communicable diseases is beyond the scope of this guide and is not the focus of this chapter. Instead, the chapters in this part of the guide are intended to serve as an overview of how certain infection-control principles traditionally used to prevent client infections can help to control infectious disease hazards for all. The caregiver is cautioned that the chapters in this section are not intended to be a comprehensive infection-control reference. Caregivers are encouraged to consult their facility's infection-control and employee-health policies for disease-prevention guidance specific to their practice setting.

DISEASE TRANSMISSION IN HEALTH CARE

Health care–associated infections (HAIs) are infections acquired by clients during the course of receiving treatment for other conditions or by caregivers during care delivery.

Certain conditions must be met for disease transmission. A **reservoir**—a place (object, animal, or human) where pathogens can thrive—is necessary. There must be a pathway out of, or away from, the reservoir, typically called a **portal of exit.** The mechanism of transfer of the pathogen is called the **mode of transmission.** For transmission to occur, there must be an unprotected **portal of entry,** or route of entry into the body. Even then, the pathogen will cause disease only in a **susceptible host**—a person who cannot defend against infection from a pathogen. These individuals lack sufficient immune capability to resist disease.

THE CHAIN OF INFECTION

In the **chain of infection,** applicable to any communicable disease, the elements required for disease transmission are represented by sequential links in a chain. Each link must be present and intact for disease transmission to occur. These links are described in the following paragraphs. (See Figure 8-1.)

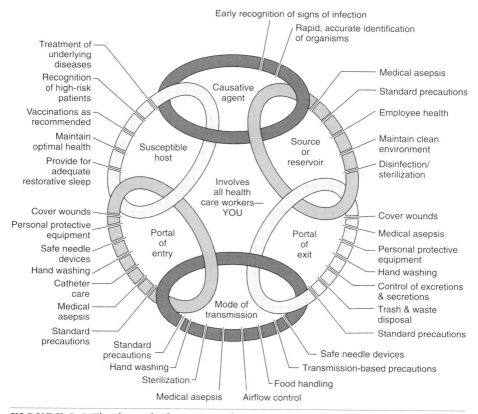

FIGURE 8-1 *The chain of infection is similar to any chain—if one link is broken, the infection cannot be spread. Shown here are the chain of infection with examples of the ways caregivers can break each link to prevent disease transmission.*

Pathogen

For disease to occur, the quantity, frequency, and duration of exposure to the pathogen must be sufficient to produce disease. Quantity is related to the volume of secretions or body fluid involved in the unprotected exposure and the concentration of the pathogen in the secretion or body fluid. Frequent unprotected exposures of long duration increase the exposure dose.

Reservoir

A reservoir is simply a place where pathogens can thrive. It may be a living creature or an object. Caregivers should assume that all human body fluids are infectious and control exposure accordingly.

Food is also a potential reservoir for pathogens in health care. Perishable foods should be discarded after 2 hours at room temperature (the **two-hour rule**), or after 1 hour if air temperatures exceed 90°F. Food should not be eaten (or stored) in client-care areas or specimen-preparation areas.

Portal of Exit

The portal of exit is the pathogen's pathway out of, or away from, the reservoir. Pathogens typically exit the human body through body fluids.

Mode of Transmission

The mode of transmission is the way in which the pathogen is passed—the pathogen's method of transfer or travel once it has exited the reservoir. Contact, droplet, and airborne modes of transmission are the most significant in the health care setting.

Contact Transmission

Most pathogens are spread through direct or indirect contact. **Direct contact** occurs when virulent pathogens are transferred directly from the reservoir to the susceptible host. **Indirect contact** typically occurs when pathogens are transferred from the reservoir to equipment or to a surface (including hands) that then comes into contact with the susceptible host.

Droplet Transmission

Droplet transmission is a form of direct contact transmission that occurs when pathogens contained in **aerosolized** body fluids (fluids that have been converted into a fine spray) are transferred directly from the reservoir to the mucous membranes of a susceptible host. These larger droplets rapidly settle out of the air, typically landing on surfaces within about a 3-foot radius, which may include the mucous membranes of the susceptible host's eyes, nose, or mouth. When produced and propelled by a sneeze or cough, these droplets may be smaller in size and may travel several feet.

Airborne Transmission

Airborne transmission is a form of indirect contact transmission. Pathogens spread through airborne transmission are encased in moisture droplets when they are produced; however, the droplet is smaller and dries quickly, resulting in **droplet nuclei.** Droplet nuclei are tiny particles remaining after the droplet has dried, and can float along on air currents indefinitely and may remain infectious for long periods if the air is cool and dry and is protected from direct sunlight. Droplet nuclei may infect a susceptible host distant from the infected source individual and, because of their small size, travel deeply into the lung when inhaled.

Portal of Entry

Generally, the portal of entry refers to the route of pathogen entry into a susceptible host. Chapped skin, mucous membranes, body orifices, and punctures are all potential portals of entry. **Percutaneous exposure** through a break in the skin such as a puncture from a needle or other sharp object is another potential portal of entry into the bloodstream.

Susceptible Host

Even in the event of an exposure, the pathogen will cause disease only in a susceptible host. A susceptible host is any individual who cannot defend against infection from a pathogen. Some medical treatments and medical conditions can greatly amplify the risk of infectious disease. Individuals with dangerously increased vulnerability to infectious disease are said to be **immunocompromised.**

Individuals differ in their ability to fight disease. Most individuals are **immunocompetent,** with healthy, functioning immune systems that generally have the capacity to successfully defend against most pathogens.

Getting adequate rest and exercise, eating nutritious foods, and developing healthy coping strategies to reduce stress are all important to disease prevention. Immunizations are available for several serious infectious diseases; generally, such immunizations are safe and effective for most immunocompetent individuals. Immunocompromised caregivers should seek health counseling regarding work status and immunization recommendations.

Breaking the Links in the Chain of Infection

Caregivers can reduce the risk of disease transmission by using the hierarchy of controls (hazard elimination, engineering controls, administrative controls and safe work practices, and PPE) to break each link in the chain of infection. With each link that is broken, disease transmission risk is further reduced.

Introduction to the HICPAC Isolation Precautions

The two-tiered system of **isolation precautions** published by the Healthcare Infection Control Practices Advisory Committee (HICPAC) and the Centers for Disease Control and Prevention (CDC) combines engineering controls, work practice/administrative controls, and PPE to prevent infectious disease transmission. This system simultaneously targets multiple links in the chain of infection and will be discussed in later chapters.

EXPOSURE INCIDENTS

An **exposure incident** occurs when a caregiver has an unprotected encounter with a pathogen (or a hazardous chemical or substance). As in cases of injuries, exposure incidents are analyzed in an effort to discover the underlying factors contributing to the exposure so they can be addressed to prevent recurrence.

Most exposure incidents can be prevented through conscientious and consistent use of appropriate engineering and administrative controls, safe work practices, and PPE. Different hazards—and different diseases—require different controls or combinations of controls.

Reporting Exposure Incidents

Caregivers should promptly report and document exposure incidents according to their facility's policy. If the incident is not reported in a timely manner, appropriate postexposure treatment may be delayed. The caregiver may be asked to stay at home until the incubation period has passed. This policy is primarily designed to protect coworkers and clients from exposure.

Timely reporting and accurate documentation provide critical information about the exposure that may help establish the link between the source client and the caregiver illness. Unfortunately, it is often difficult to ascertain whether an illness is work related; pathogens can be transmitted in the community as well as in the health care setting, and caregivers move about freely in both environments.

Illness Monitoring

Many facilities have policies that require caregivers to report when they become ill with certain communicable diseases or conditions, even if they were not exposed to the disease at work. These reporting policies are designed to protect clients and other employees by limiting exposure to the ill caregiver. An ill caregiver may be excluded from work completely or restricted from direct care tasks until recovered. Caregivers should seek information about how these types of illnesses and absences are handled in their facility by reading the facility's policy manual or by contacting their supervisor.

CHAPTER

9

PREVENTING DISEASE TRANSMISSION—MANAGING DISEASE EXPOSURE

REGULATIONS AND GUIDELINES FOR PREVENTING DISEASE TRANSMISSION

Guidelines regarding the prevention of disease transmission may take the form of voluntary recommendations, such as practice guidelines from the Centers for Disease Control and Prevention (CDC), or mandatory regulation, such as Occupational Safety and Health Administration (OSHA) standards. Additional guidance related to communicable disease issued at the state and local health department level may be in the form of recommendations (voluntary) or regulation (compulsory). Other agencies and organizations may issue guidance as well.

HICPAC ISOLATION GUIDELINES

The two-tiered system of isolation precautions developed by the CDC and the Healthcare Infection Control Practices Advisory Committee (HICPAC) includes standard precautions and transmission-based precautions (airborne, droplet, and contact). These precautions are used in conjunction with a table of selected infections and recommended precautions found on the CDC

Web site. (Consult the text on which this guide is based, *Working Safely in Health Care, A Practical Guide,* for additional information on accessing information from the CDC Web site.) Each category of precautions prescribes unique combinations of engineering, administrative and safe work-practice controls, and personal protective equipment (PPE) based on the mode of pathogen transmission.

It is important to use the correct PPE based on an organism's known mode of transmission. PPE that is intended for use in preventing or treating disease is subject to regulation by the **Food and Drug Administration Center for Devices and Radiological Health (FDA CDRH),** a federal agency within the U.S. Department of Health and Human Services that is responsible for ensuring the safety and effectiveness of medical devices and eliminating unnecessary human exposure to man-made radiation from medical, occupational, and consumer products.

The four categories of precautions are discussed in the following paragraphs and are summarized in Table 9-1.

TABLE 9-1   Summary of Types of Precautions

	Standard Precautions	Airborne Precautions	Droplet Precautions	Contact Precautions
Applicability	Apply to blood, all body fluids, secretions, and excretions except sweat, regardless of whether they contain visible blood, nonintact skin, and mucous membranes. Apply to all clients with known or unknown diagnoses; designed to reduce the risk of transmission of pathogens from diagnosed and undiagnosed sources of infection.	In addition to Standard Precautions. Apply to clients having known or suspected serious illnesses transmitted by airborne droplet nuclei (e.g., active pulmonary tuberculosis, varicella, measles).	In addition to Standard Precautions. Apply to clients known or suspected to have illnesses transmitted by large particle droplets (e.g., seasonal influenza, pertussis, *Neisseria meningitidis*).	In addition to Standard Precautions. Apply to clients having known or suspected serious illnesses transmitted by direct or indirect contact (e.g., wound infections, varicella, *Clostridium difficile*).
Character of organism	Pathogens thriving on moist body surfaces and in blood and other body fluids	Five microns or smaller in size. May remain suspended in the air for long periods of time	Typically >5 microns in size. Direct contact with mucous membranes of eyes, nose, or mouth	Pathogens invading wounds or lesions or infecting gastrointestinal tract

(continued)

TABLE 9-1   (continued)

	Standard Precautions	Airborne Precautions	Droplet Precautions	Contact Precautions
Administrative and safe work-practice controls	Hand washing and antisepsis, use of safe needle devices and other measures to prevent sharps injuries, prompt cleanup of spills, appropriate handling of all waste materials, adequate housekeeping procedures for cleaning and disinfection of surfaces, and thoughtful selection of client room placement. Clients who may contaminate the environment should be placed in a private room whenever possible.	In addition to Standard Precautions: surgical mask on client when outside room. Private room, with door kept closed at all times. Observation to ensure that ventilation system is functioning.	In addition to Standard Precautions: private room if possible. Maintain 3-foot or greater distance from client if PPE is not worn. Surgical mask on client when outside room. Cough etiquette.	In addition to Standard Precautions: private room if possible. Contact precautions require the use of nonsterile gloves when entering the client's room. Should a client need to be moved from the room, care should be taken to maintain precautions to minimize exposure to others and to prevent contamination of environmental surfaces.
PPE*	Use of PPE when handling blood and body fluids, touching client equipment and soiled linens. Chosen based on the task at hand. Examples include gloves, surgical mask, eye protection, and gowns.	In addition to Standard Precautions: properly fitted NIOSH-approved air-purifying filtering respirator, N-95 minimum.	In addition to Standard Precautions: surgical mask to protect mucous membranes of nose and mouth. *Best practice: protect mucous membranes of eyes.*	In addition to Standard Precautions: gloves donned when entering room. If direct client contact or contact with potentially contaminated items in the room is anticipated, a nonsterile gown should be donned upon entering the room.
Engineering Controls (Mechanical equipment)	Not required	Special ventilation required	Not required. Unless in a spray, droplets typically do not carry far in the air, up to 3 feet.	Not required

PPE that is intended for use in preventing or treating disease is subject to regulation under the device provisions of the Federal Food, Drug, and Cosmetic Act. This includes surgical masks, surgical N-95 respirators, medical gloves, and surgical gowns.

Note: This table is not intended to reflect all aspects of each category of precautions, but is representative of controls that fall under a specific precaution.

Source: Adapted from HICPAC Isolation Precautions for Hospitals, http://www.cdc.gov/ncidod/dhqp/gl_isolation.html.

Standard Precautions

Standard precautions expanded the concept of universal precautions, which applied only to blood and other potentially infectious material as defined by OSHA (OPIM), to include all body fluids except sweat (regardless of whether visible blood was present), nonintact skin, and mucous membranes. Controls for both include using safe needle devices, proper disposal of contaminated items, use of PPE, and rigorous hand hygiene. See Figure 9-1.

STANDARD PRECAUTIONS
FOR INFECTION CONTROL

Wash Hands (Plain soap)
Wash after touching **blood, body fluids, secretions, excretions,** and **contaminated items.** Wash immediately **after gloves are removed** and **between patient contacts.** Avoid transfer of microorganisms to other patients or environments.

Wear Gloves
Wear when touching **blood, body fluids, secretions, excretions,** and **contaminated items.** Put on **clean** gloves just **before touching mucous membranes** and **nonintact skin.** Change gloves between tasks and procedures on the same patient after contact with material that may contain high concentrations of microorganisms. Remove gloves promptly after use, before touching noncontaminated items and environmental surfaces, and before going to another patient, and wash hands immediately to avoid transfer of microorganisms to other patients or environments.

Wear Mask and Eye Protection or Face Shield
Protect mucous membranes of the eyes, nose, and mouth during procedures and patient-care activities that are likely to generate **splashes** or **sprays** of **blood, body fluids, secretions,** or **excretions.**

Wear Gown
Protect skin and prevent soiling of clothing during procedures that are likely to generate **splashes** or **sprays** of **blood, body fluids, secretions,** or **excretions.** Remove a soiled gown as promptly as possible and wash hands to avoid transfer of microorganisms to other patients or environments.

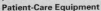

Patient-Care Equipment
Handle used patient-care equipment soiled with **blood, body fluids, secretions,** or **excretions** in a manner that prevents skin and mucous membrane exposures, contamination of clothing, and transfer of microorganisms to other patients and environments. Ensure that reusable equipment is not used for the care of another patient until it has been appropriately cleaned and reprocessed and single-use items are properly discarded.

Environmental Control
Follow hospital procedures for routine care, cleaning, and disinfection of environmental surfaces, beds, bed rails, bedside equipment, and other frequently touched surfaces.

Linen
Handle, transport, and process used linen soiled with **blood, body fluids, secretions,** or **excretions** in a manner that prevents exposures and contamination of clothing, and avoids transfer of microorganisms to other patients and environments.

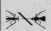
Occupational Health and Bloodborne Pathogens
Use safe needle devices and other safe sharps. Prevent injuries when using needles, scalpels, and other sharp instruments or devices; when handling sharp instruments after procedures; when cleaning used instruments; and when disposing of used needles.

Never recap used needles using both hands or any other technique that involves directing the point of a needle toward any part of the body; rather, use either a one-handed "scoop" technique or a mechanical device designed for holding the needle sheath.

Do not remove needles from disposable syringes by hand, and do not bend, break, or otherwise manipulate used needles by hand. Place used disposable syringes and needles, scalpel blades, and other sharp items in puncture-resistant sharps containers located as close as practical to the area in which the items were used, and place reusable syringes and needles in a puncture-resistant container for transport to the reprocessing area.

Use **resuscitation devices** as an alternative to mouth-to-mouth resuscitation.

Patient Placement
Use a **private room** for a patient who contaminates the environment or who does not (or cannot be expected to) assist in maintaining appropriate hygiene or environmental control. Consult Infection Control if a private room is not available.

FIGURE 9-1 Standard Precautions for Infection Control issued by the CDC. *(Courtesy of the Brevis Corporation.)*

Hand Hygiene in Standard Precautions

Hand hygiene is the most important control in standard precautions. **Hand hygiene** is a general term that includes activities directed at preventing disease transmission via the hands. Hand cleansing, skin care, nail care, and avoiding the use of artificial nails are all important aspects of hand hygiene. Hand hygiene is indicated before client contact and before donning gloves, after touching intact or nonintact client skin, mucous membranes, wounds and dressings, and body fluids or excretions. Hand hygiene is also indicated after removing gloves. Nails should be kept clean and short. Skin should be kept in good condition by using facility-approved lotions provided in pump containers.

Caregivers should promptly report skin problems to the supervisor. Skin problems can become serious and may require medical attention if ignored.

Latex Exposure to latex may result in allergic reactions in some individuals. (See Figure 9-2.) Used properly, latex gloves have proved effective in preventing transmission of many infectious diseases and may be safely used by most caregivers. Concerns about exposure to latex products should be promptly brought to the attention of the supervisor.

Additional Controls in Standard Precautions

Standard precautions also include the prompt cleanup of spills, appropriate handling of all waste materials, use of safe needle devices, sharps containers, and other measures to prevent sharps injuries, disinfection procedures, and thoughtful selection of client room placement.

PPE selection in standard precautions is task specific; if a procedure could potentially result in a splash to the mucous membranes of the eye or nose, PPE should be selected to protect those portals of entry. Standard precautions should be practiced by all caregivers at all times, regardless of client diagnosis. Additional information on PPE is presented later in this chapter.

Transmission-Based Precautions

Airborne, droplet, and contact precautions are always used in conjunction with standard precautions. Diseases and appropriate precautions can be found in the table at Appendix A of the Guideline for Isolation Precautions in Hospitals posted on the CDC Web site. The use of multiple precautions may be necessary when agents can be transmitted through more than one mode.

Airborne Precautions

Airborne precautions are used in addition to standard precautions for those clients with known or suspected diagnosis of a disease transmitted via the airborne route. These pathogens may be encased in tiny droplet nuclei that

*N*IOSH
ALERT

Preventing Allergic Reactions
to Natural Rubber Latex in the Workplace

WARNING!

Workers exposed to latex gloves and other products containing natural rubber latex may develop allergic reactions such as skin rashes; hives; nasal, eye, or sinus symptoms; asthma; and (rarely) shock.

Workers with ongoing exposure to natural rubber latex* should take the following steps to protect themselves:

1. Use nonlatex gloves for activities that are not likely to involve contact with infectious materials (food preparation, routine housekeeping, maintenance, etc.).

2. Appropriate barrier protection is necessary when handling infectious materials.[†] If you choose latex gloves, use powder-free gloves with reduced protein content.[‡]

3. When wearing latex gloves, do not use oil-based hand creams or lotions (which can cause glove deterioration) unless they have been shown to reduce latex-related problems and maintain glove barrier protection.

4. Frequently clean work areas contaminated with latex dust (upholstery, carpets, ventilation ducts, and plenums).

5. Frequently change the ventilation filters and vacuum bags used in latex-contaminated areas.

6. Learn to recognize the symptoms of latex allergy: skin rashes; hives; flushing; itching; nasal, eye, or sinus symptoms; asthma; and shock.

7. If you develop symptoms of latex allergy, avoid direct contact with latex gloves and products until you can see a physician experienced in treating latex allergy.

8. If you have latex allergy, consult your physician regarding the following precautions:

    • Avoid contact with latex gloves and products.
    • Avoid areas where you might inhale the powder from the latex gloves worn by others.
    • Tell your employers, physicians, nurses, and dentists that you have latex allergy.
    • Wear a medical alert bracelet.

9. Take advantage of all latex allergy education and training provided by your employer.

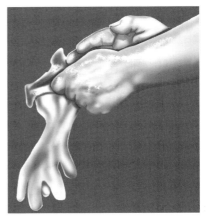

Dust produced by removing a latex glove containing powder.

---

* In this warning sheet, the term "latex" refers to natural rubber latex and includes products made from dry natural rubber. Natural rubber latex is the product manufactured from a milky fluid derived mainly from the rubber tree, *Hevea brasiliensis*.
[†]CDC (Centers for Disease Control and Prevention) [1987]. Recommendations for prevention of HIV transmission in healthcare settings. MMWR *36*(S2).
[‡]The goal of this recommendation is to reduce exposure to allergy-causing proteins (antigens). Until well-accepted standardized tests are available, total protein serves as a useful indicator of the exposure of concern.

FIGURE 9-2 *The National Institute for Occupational Safety and Health (NIOSH) has provided information to warn caregivers about the hazards of latex products. (Department of Health and Human Services [NIOSH] Publication No. 97-135.)*

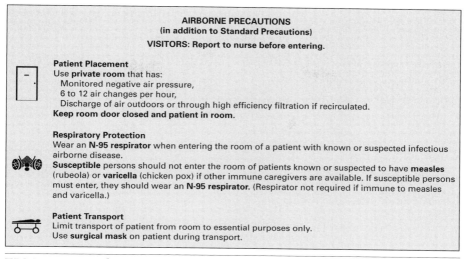

AIRBORNE PRECAUTIONS
(in addition to Standard Precautions)
VISITORS: Report to nurse before entering.

Patient Placement
Use **private room** that has:
  Monitored negative air pressure,
  6 to 12 air changes per hour,
  Discharge of air outdoors or through high efficiency filtration if recirculated.
Keep room door closed and patient in room.

Respiratory Protection
Wear an **N-95 respirator** when entering the room of a patient with known or suspected infectious airborne disease.
Susceptible persons should not enter the room of patients known or suspected to have **measles** (rubeola) or **varicella** (chicken pox) if other immune caregivers are available. If susceptible persons must enter, they should wear an **N-95 respirator**. (Respirator not required if immune to measles and varicella.)

Patient Transport
Limit transport of patient from room to essential purposes only.
Use **surgical mask** on patient during transport.

FIGURE 9-4 Airborne precautions, one category of transmission-based precautions.

become airborne on release from the client reservoir and may remain airborne for extended periods, traveling great distances. (See Figure 9-4.)

Airborne precautions recommend client placement in a private, **negative pressure room**—one in which the exhaust airflow is designed to prevent contaminated air in the client room from flowing into adjacent areas. The system is not effective unless the door is kept closed and the system is turned on. Most facilities have a visual indicator such as a gauge to indicate that the system is on.

In addition to the special airflow requirements of a negative pressure room, airborne precautions require caregivers to wear **air-purifying respirators** designed to serve as a barrier to protect the caregiver airway from airborne pathogens. Air is drawn through filtering devices to remove contaminants from the air before it is inhaled.

Air-purifying respirators come in many types and are selected based on the type of airborne hazard. Most individuals can wear a respirator safely, but as a precaution, OSHA requires that caregivers be cleared by a medical professional before a respirator can be worn. Hooded respirators do not have to fit snugly. They are often a good alternative for individuals who cannot physically tolerate a tight-fitting respirator.

Air-purifying respirators commonly used in airborne precautions are called **N-95 respirators.** An N-95 respirator is an air-purifying filtering respirator that is designed to remove 95% of particles (i.e., microbes) of 0.3 microns in size from the air before it is inhaled. The N-95 respirator protects only against particles and is the minimally accepted caregiver protection for use in airborne precautions. Respirators are discussed in more detail in the PPE section of this chapter.

Client Transport and Outpatient Settings

If client transport is necessary, it is recommended that a surgical mask (not a respirator) be placed on the client to capture the moisture droplets. Limit transport outside the negative pressure room. In situations where there may be contact with others, scheduling during less crowded times, and perhaps using alternative entrances, can help to reduce transmission risk.

Droplet Precautions

Droplet precautions are used in addition to standard precautions for those clients with known or suspected diagnosis of a disease transmitted via the droplet route. They are summarized in Figure 9-5. Although generally too small to see with the naked eye, the large size causes the droplets to rapidly settle out of the air, typically landing on surfaces within about a 3-foot radius of the client, which may include the mucous membranes of the caregiver's eyes, nose, or mouth. When propelled by a sneeze or cough, these droplets may travel several feet.

In addition to standard precautions, caregivers should wear a surgical mask when providing care within 3 feet of the client. Although not specified in the guidelines at the time of this writing, eye protection is a good idea when caring for these clients, as the mucous membrane of the eye is a potential portal of entry for these pathogens. For tasks outside this 3-foot radius, standard precautions are considered adequate and a surgical mask is not recommended.

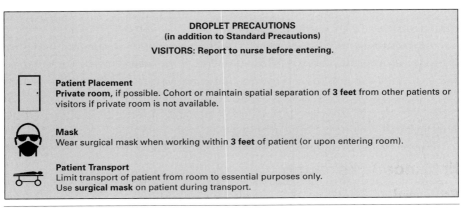

FIGURE 9-5 Droplet precautions, one category of transmission-based precautions.

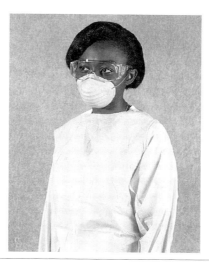

FIGURE 9-6 An example of a surgical mask. *A surgical mask protects the mucous membranes of the mouth and nose from direct contact with droplets containing pathogens. Close-fitting safety glasses or goggles protect the eyes. A surgical mask is different from a respirator.*

Ideally, these clients should be placed in a private room. Special engineering controls are not required for droplet precautions, and the door does not need to remain closed.

Client Transport and Outpatient Settings

Consideration for managing client transport and outpatient settings is similar to that of airborne precautions.

Contact Precautions

Contact precautions are used in addition to standard precautions for clients with a wound or other infection known or suspected to be caused by a pathogen transmitted via the contact route.

Contact precautions require the use of nonsterile gloves when entering the client's room. This differs from standard precautions, for which glove use is task dependent. Such clients should be placed in private rooms or in rooms where other clients have the same infectious condition. (See Figure 9-7.)

Enhanced Precautions

Enhanced precautions were developed for pathogens that may be transmitted by all modes of transmission or for which transmission route is

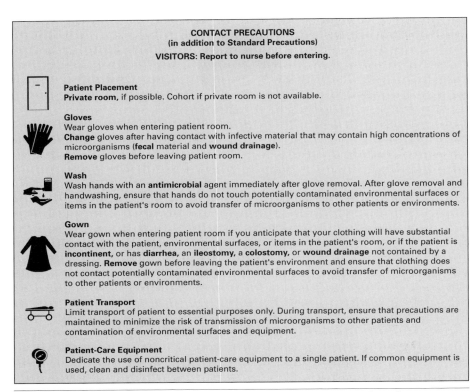

FIGURE 9-7 Contact precautions, one category of transmission-based precautions.

unknown. Enhanced precautions consist of all four categories of precautions (standard, airborne, droplet, and contact) used in combination, in addition to eye protection when within 3 feet of the client.

ISOLATION PRECAUTIONS FOR SPECIFIC INFECTIONS

The CDC offers many online resources for the caregiver on its Web site, including a detailed definition for each category of precautions. The Web site also provides a reference that specifically details which type of isolation precaution is appropriate for more than 200 pathogens. An example of the type of information provided can be found in Table 9-2. This Web site is also an excellent resource for information on pathogens that may be responsible for emerging diseases. Consult the text on which this guide is based, *Working Safely in Health Care, A Practical Guide,* for information on accessing this information from the CDC Web site.

TABLE 9-2 Example of Information Found at Appendix A: Type and Duration of Precautions Needed for Selected Infections and Conditions

Infection/Condition	Precaution	
	Type*	Duration**
Abscess, draining, major	C	DI
Conjunctivitis, acute bacterial	S	
Gastroenteritis, *C. difficile*	C	DI
HIV	S	
Influenza	D	DI
Tuberculosis, pulmonary	A	F
Whooping cough (pertussis)	D	F

*A = airborne; C = contact; D = droplet; S = standard.

**DI = duration of illness; U = time specified in hours; F = see footnote in Appendix A.

Source: Excerpted and adapted from Appendix A, Guideline for Isolation Precautions in Hospitals, http://www.cdc.gov/ncidod/dhqp/gl_isolation_appendixA.html

PERSONAL PROTECTIVE EQUIPMENT FOR THE PREVENTION OF DISEASE TRANSMISSION

PPE includes protective clothing and equipment such as gowns, gloves, goggles, face shields, surgical masks, and respirators. Everyday work clothes are not considered PPE. Proper PPE selection, maintenance, and use is critical to preventing disease transmission. Employers should provide appropriate PPE at no cost to the caregiver. It should be properly fitted, and the caregiver should be thoroughly trained in its use.

Protective Clothing

Selection of protective clothing is based on the task and may range from a cotton gown to an impermeable gown or apron with protective booties. It is essential that PPE be removed before the caregiver leaves the immediate work area.

Glove Considerations

Hand hygiene and appropriate selection and use of gloves are essential in preventing disease transmission. Gloves do not provide complete protection; pathogens may enter through defects in the gloves, and contamination may occur during glove removal. Hand cleansing is still necessary.

Gloves used to prevent disease transmission are typically made of natural rubber latex or synthetic materials such as vinyl and nitrile. The protection afforded by a glove varies based on quality of glove material, duration and intensity of use, and manufacturer.

Gloves that are appropriate to protect against pathogens may not be appropriate protection when using disinfectants or other chemicals. Always consult the material data safety sheet (MSDS) if you are unsure. Hands should always be cleansed after glove removal.

Respiratory Protection in Airborne Precautions

Respiratory protection is a type of PPE essential to the prevention of airborne disease transmission. There are many types of respirators, but all provide a barrier between the airborne contaminant and the caregiver's airway, or portal of entry. The discussion of respiratory protection in this guide will be limited to the types of respirators most commonly used in health care for the prevention of airborne disease transmission. All respirators approved for use in the workplace must undergo rigorous testing, be approved by NIOSH, and display the NIOSH approval logo. In addition, respirators intended for use in preventing or treating disease must *also* be evaluated for flammability and fluid resistance and approved by the FDA CDRH. For prevention of disease transmission, respiratory protection should be used in the context of precautions prescribed in the HICPAC Guideline for Isolation Precautions in Hospitals.

Air-Purifying Respirators

Most air-purifying respirators are **negative pressure respirators.** Negative pressure respirators have a face-piece that fits snugly and seals with the face. Negative pressure air-purifying respirators require users to draw air through the air-purifying cartridge or filter as they inhale, which may take considerable cardiovascular effort.

Negative pressure air-purifying respirators are lightweight and convenient to use. However, they do not supply oxygen and must be selected based on hazard and fit.

Disposable negative pressure air-purifying filtering face-piece respirators are most commonly used for the prevention of disease transmission in health care. An example of this type of respirator can be found in Figure 9-10c. These filtering face-piece respirators remove particles from the air before the air is inhaled; they do not remove vapors or gases. Other types of respirators are used for protection against other types of airborne contaminants. Questions about respirators for other tasks should be directed to the safety professional.

N-95 Respirator   The disposable negative pressure filtering face-piece respirator (N-95 respirator) is the minimal respiratory protection prescribed for airborne precautions. It is typically made of a fluid-resistant fibrous material,

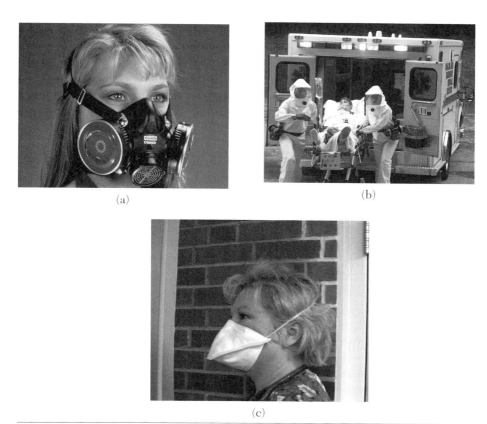

FIGURE 9-10 Examples of air-purifying respirators. *(a) An example of a negative pressure air-purifying respirator with removable cartridges. This respirator is more commonly seen in industrial settings and is not approved for use in direct client care. Courtesy of Mine Safety Appliances (MSA) Company North America (888) MSA-2222. (b) An example of a powered air-purifying respirator. The powered air-purifying respirator is commonly used in areas where risk of airborne disease transmission is high, such as bronchoscopy and similar procedures on clients with suspected or confirmed airborne disease diagnoses. Courtesy of Mine Safety Appliances (MSA) Company North America (888) MSA-2222. (c) An example of an N-95 filtering face-piece respirator. This type of respirator is the most widely used in the acute-care setting. To provide adequate protection, it must be specially fitted to each caregiver. Notice how the straps are placed to provide a snug fit.*

held snugly to the caregiver's face with elastic bands. An example is provided in Figure 9-10c. "N-95" describes the filter efficiency rating generally accepted as minimal protection for use in airborne precautions.

N-95 disposable air-purifying respirators serve a distinctly different purpose from surgical masks. In addition to splash protection, these respirators protect the caregiver airway from tiny airborne particles. In contrast, surgical masks protect the mucous membranes of the nose and mouth from direct contact with splashes and larger droplets or particles. Surgical masks are not respirators and do not purify the air.

Disposable N-95 respirators are most commonly used in airborne precautions but sometimes present great challenges to a good fit. Even when the fit is good, they do not fit as tightly as do other types, which can reduce the protection they offer. Larger particles can be inhaled around the edges of the respirator. Because of the looser fit, they are not the best choice for environments where substances are unknown or their concentrations are high. Additional protection may also be recommended for certain procedures or when caring for clients infected with especially virulent pathogens.

Powered air-purifying respirators may be used when negative pressure masks are inadequate or unavailable or facial features prohibit a good face seal. They are recommended during cough induction and when other aerosol-generating procedures are conducted with clients known or suspected to have an infectious disease that may be transmitted by the airborne route.

Consult the text on which this guide is based, *Working Safely in Health Care, A Practical Guide,* for additional information related to respiratory protection.

Medical Clearance for Respirator Use

The OSHA respirator medical evaluation is required prior to respirator use. The evaluation is certification that the user is medically fit to wear a respirator. Medical history, current medical conditions, and smoking habits are all important considerations. Some medical conditions may preclude caregivers from wearing respirators because respirators cause such an increased workload on the heart and lungs.

Respirator Fit-Testing

Respirator fit-testing is done annually by qualified personnel using protocols established and mandated by OSHA to ensure a properly fitting respirator. A properly fitting respirator provides the greatest protection from respiratory hazards. Without fit-testing, caregivers cannot be sure that the respirator fits properly and is protecting them.

The fit-testing process is not to be confused with the **user seal check** required each time a respirator is donned to see if the face-piece is properly seated. Different manufacturers may prescribe a slightly different user seal check procedure. If the caregiver is unable to complete the user seal check successfully, the seal is likely not adequate and the caregiver should avoid exposure to clients who may be infected with airborne disease until another complete fit-test is performed.

Additional Administrative and Safe Work-Practice Controls

When hands are visibly soiled, they should be washed with soap and water for a minimum of 15 seconds. If hands are not visibly soiled, alcohol-based hand disinfectants may be used. Care should be given to work the cleaner into all areas of the hand to include the nail beds and to rub the cleaner on hands until completely dry.

Health Screening

A baseline health inventory is often used shortly after hire to assess caregivers for known infectious diseases, immunization status, and medical conditions that could predispose them to acquire or transmit a communicable disease. Screening recommendations are posted on the CDC Web site, and state and local health departments may require specific additional screening. These screenings may be repeated at intervals.

Most organizations routinely screen for immunity to certain vaccine-preventable diseases. Additional screenings using laboratory analysis of blood counts, urinalysis, and other testing have not been established as either beneficial or cost effective.

Control of Disease through Immunizations

Immunizations are an important element of preventing disease transmission. The CDC periodically publishes recommendations for caregiver immunizations. (See Table 9-3.)

Immunization is an effective control to prevent hepatitis B transmission. OSHA requires that the hepatitis B vaccine be offered at no charge to employees who may encounter workplace exposure to bloodborne pathogens, but it cannot be required.

Employee health professionals have expertise to evaluate an exposure and manage **postexposure prophylaxis (PEP).** Postexposure prophylaxis is medical treatment provided to prevent disease and is generally pathogen-specific. See Table 9-4 for examples of postexposure immunizations. Employee health professionals typically coordinate with infection-control professionals to assist with the control of further exposures. Work restrictions may be necessary to protect others from the caregiver or to protect the caregiver from others with an infectious condition. Table 9-5 lists examples of suggested caregiver work restrictions. Exposure incidents that result in disease transmission may be covered under workers' compensation.

TABLE 9-3 Recommended Immunizations for Health Care Workers*

Hepatitis B	Two doses intramuscularly (IM) 4 weeks apart, third dose 5 months after second dose; booster doses not necessary.
Influenza	Annual vaccination with current vaccine, IM.
Measles	One dose subcutaneously (SC); second dose at least 1 month later. Vaccination should be considered for all health care workers who lack proof of immunity, including those born before 1957.
Mumps	Routine vaccination of health care workers: persons born during or after 1957 without other evidence of immunity: two doses of a live mumps virus vaccine SC (second dose at least 1 month after first). Vaccination of health care workers born before 1957; consider one dose of live mumps virus vaccine if there is no other evidence of immunity.
Rubella	One dose, SC, no booster.
Varicella–zoster	Two doses SC 4 to 8 weeks apart if ≥13 years of age.

*Refer to CDC guidelines for updated guidance, a more detailed explanation of vaccination indications, major precautions and contraindications, and special considerations.

Source: Excerpt adapted from Table 2. Immunizing Agents and Immunization Schedules for Health-care Workers (HCWs) in Immunization of Health-Care Workers: Recommendations of the Advisory Committee on Immunization Practices (ACIP) and the Hospital Infection Control Practices Advisory Committee (HICPAC) (December 26, 1997) and Updated Recommendations of the Advisory Committee on Immunization Practices (ACIP) for the Control and Elimination of Mumps (June 1, 2006).

TABLE 9-4 Examples of Postexposure Recommended Immunizations for Nonimmune Employees

Hepatitis B immune globulin (HBIG)	Postexposure prophylaxis. Administer as soon as possible after exposure (but no later than 7 days after exposure). A second dose of HBIG should be administered 1 month after if the hepatitis B vaccination series has not been started.
Varicella–zoster immune globulin (VZIG)	Recommended for persons known or likely to be susceptible who have close and prolonged exposure to a contact case or to an infectious hospital staff worker or client.

Source: CDC recommendations for immunization of health care workers, Postexposure. Excerpt adapted from Table 2, Immunizing Agents Strongly Recommended for Health Care Workers, www.cdc.gov/mmwr/preview/mmwrhtml/00050577.htm#00002863.htm.

TABLE 9-5   Recommended Work Restrictions for Caregivers with Possible Infectious Diseases

Disease	Work Restriction	Duration
Conjunctivitis	Restrict from client contact and contact with client environment	Until discharge ceases
Diarrhea, acute	Restrict from client contact, contact with client environment, and food handling	Until symptoms resolve
Hepatitis A	Restrict from client contact, contact with client environment, and food handling	Until 7 days after onset of jaundice
Hepatitis B, acute or chronic, in health care workers who perform invasive procedures	Do not perform exposure-prone invasive procedures until counsel from an expert review panel has been sought. Refer to state regulations	Until hepatitis B e antigen is negative.
Hepatitis B, acute or chronic, in health care workers who do not perform exposure-prone procedures	No restrictions beyond standard precautions	
Hepatitis C	No recommendation (unresolved issue)	
Herpes simplex		
Genital	No restriction	
Hands (herpetic whitlow)	Restrict from client contact and contact with the client environment	Until lesions heal
Orofacial	Evaluate for need to restrict from care of high-risk clients	
Human immunodeficiency virus (HIV)	Do not perform exposure-prone invasive procedures until counsel from an expert review panel has been sought; panel should review and recommend procedures the worker can perform, considering specific procedure as well as skill and technique of the worker; standard precautions should always be observed, refer to state guidelines	
Measles		
Active	Exclude from duty*	Until 7 days after the rash appears
Postexposure (susceptible personnel)	Exclude from duty*	From 5th day after first exposure through 21st day after last exposure and/or 4 days after rash appears

(continued)

TABLE 9-5 (continued)

Disease	Work Restriction	Duration
Meningococcal infections	Exclude from duty*	Until 24 hours after start of effective therapy
Pediculosis	Restrict from client contact	Until treated and observed to be free of adult and immature lice
Pertussis		
Active	Exclude from duty*	From beginning of catarrhal stage through 3rd week after onset of paroxysms or until 5 days after start of effective antimicrobial therapy
Postexposure (symptomatic personnel)	No restriction, prophylaxis recommended	
Postexposure (asymptomatic personnel)	Exclude from duty	Until 5 days after start of effective antimicrobial therapy
Scabies	Restrict from client contact	Until cleared by medical evaluation
Streptococcal infection, group A	Restrict from client care, contact with client environment, and food handling	Until 24 hours after adequate treatment started
Tuberculosis		
Active	Exclude from duty	Until proved noninfectious
Purified protein derivative (PPD) converter	No restriction	
Zoster		
Localized in healthy person	Cover lesions, restrict from care of high-risk clients	Until all lesions dry and crust
Generalized or localized in immunosuppressed person	Restrict from client contact	Until all lesions dry and crust
Postexposure (susceptible personnel)	Restrict from client contact	From 10th day after first exposure through 21st day (28th day if VZIG given) after last exposure or, if varicella occurs, until all lesions dry and crust
Viral respiratory infections, acute febrile	Consider excluding from the care of high-risk clients or contact with their environment during community outbreak of respiratory syncytial virus and influenza	Until acute symptoms resolve

*"Exclude from duty" should be interpreted as exclusion from the health care facility and from health care activities outside the facility.

Source: Excerpt adapted from Table 3. Summary of suggested work restrictions for health care personnel exposed to or infected with infectious diseases of importance in health care settings, in the absence of state and local regulations (modified from ACIP recommendations) in Guidelines for Infection Control in Health Care Personnel, 1998. Centers for Disease Control and Prevention.

CHAPTER

10

BLOODBORNE DISEASE PREVENTION AND SHARPS SAFETY

INTRODUCTION

The Occupational Safety and Health Administration (OSHA) published the Bloodborne Pathogens Standard (29 CFR 1910.1030) in 1991 in an effort to prevent transmission of bloodborne pathogens (BBPs). In November 2000, the passage of the Needlestick Safety and Prevention Act prompted a revision of the standard. This chapter will highlight the main worker protections afforded by these laws.

Although other diseases may be carried and transmitted through the blood and other potentially infectious materials (OPIM), the human immunodeficiency virus (HIV), hepatitis B virus (HBV), and hepatitis C virus (HCV) are the focus of the OSHA Bloodborne Pathogen Standard and will be the focus of this chapter. These pathogens may be transmitted as a result of events that compromise skin integrity, such as percutaneous exposures and chapped skin, and transmission occurs more frequently when the exposure incident involves visible blood. Increased risk for disease transmission is associated with larger-bore needles and deeper wounds than with more superficial injuries. OSHA requires that, regardless of the injury, all BBP exposure incidents be reported according to facility policy.

TRANSMISSION OF BLOODBORNE PATHOGENS

The OSHA rule brought about significant changes in isolation practices, mandating the use of universal precautions for contact with blood and OPIM. With the development of the Healthcare Infection Control Practices Advisory Committee (HICPAC) Isolation Precautions in 1996, universal precautions were expanded to the standard precautions in use at the time of this writing. The OSHA rule has not been changed, however, and still uses the universal precautions terminology.

Transmission of bloodborne pathogens occurs most easily through exposure to infectious blood and body fluids containing visible blood. Although OPIM may contain bloodborne pathogens, the actual rate of transmission is considerably less when not in the presence of blood. Unless visible blood is present, feces, nasal secretions, saliva, sputum, tears, urine, and vomitus are highly unlikely to transmit *bloodborne* disease, such as HBV, HCV, and HIV. The caregiver should not misinterpret this to mean that these other body fluids do not contain pathogens and cannot transmit disease. They do and they can. Because of that, standard precautions are required for all body fluids, except sweat.

Bloodborne pathogens are transmitted most often through percutaneous exposures. The activities most commonly associated with percutaneous injury are two-handed recapping of a used needle and disposal of the sharp into a receptacle.

The risk associated with transmission of bloodborne pathogens is influenced by the source client disease status—that is, whether or not the source client is infected with a bloodborne pathogen. This is not always known at the time of the exposure incident. If the source client is infected, the risk of transmission is influenced by the virulence of the pathogen involved in the exposure incident, the depth of the wound, the amount of blood involved, the presence of visible blood on the device involved in the incident, and whether the device is hollow-bore and has been used in an artery or vein. Risk also depends on the **viral load** of the source client, which is basically the amount, or concentration, of virus in the source client's blood. For example, a client who has just recently **seroconverted,** or changed from a noninfected state to an infected state, will have a lower viral load, so may be less likely to transmit a disease than a client at the end stage of an infectious disease process.

The employer has an obligation under the OSHA Bloodborne Pathogen Standard to provide a medical evaluation in the event of an occupational exposure incident involving blood or OPIM. This evaluation may be done by the facility Employee Health Service or another provider. Either way, this evaluation is important in determining the severity of the exposure and guiding postexposure prophylaxis and medical-management decisions.

Transmission Risk

In general, the risk of transmission from an infected client to a health care worker is approximately 3 to 10% for HBV, 3% for HCV, 0.3% for HIV for a percutaneous exposure, and 0.09% for HIV for a mucous membrane exposure. Transmission of HIV from a nonintact skin exposure has not been well quantified but is believed to be less than mucous membrane exposures.

The Needlestick Safety and Prevention Act

This Act, passed in November 2000, implemented a change to the Bloodborne Pathogens Standard, 29 CFR 1910.1030 in response to continuing high rates of exposure to bloodborne pathogens by health care personnel. The Act made it necessary for employers to take an active role in the identification, evaluation, and implementation of the use of safer medical devices. It required additional record-keeping requirements specific to sharps injuries. Some of the changes include sharps disposal containers, self-sheathing needles, and safer medical devices such as needleless devices. Caregivers who use these devices should participate in the selection of new products.

Effective Use of the Hierarchy of Controls to Prevent BBP Transmission

More stringent than OSHA rules, consistent and conscientious use of engineering, administrative, and PPE controls incorporated into the HICPAC Isolation Precautions introduced in previous chapters will significantly reduce the risk of infection in the event of an exposure incident.

Knowing the nature of the exposure helps to assess risk of actual disease transmission. Whether disease will result from an exposure incident is dependent on the pathogen involved and the viral load of the source client, the amount of source blood involved in the exposure, the type of exposure suffered (i.e., a deep laceration with a scalpel versus a superficial wound from an insulin syringe), and the individual health of the exposed individual, including immunity status.

One of the best ways to reduce potential needle-stick injuries is to eliminate unnecessary injections through the use of needleless devices and increased use of oral medications rather than percutaneous or intravenous (IV) routes when clinically feasible. When the injection cannot be eliminated, use of safe needle devices is an effective engineering control. An example of such a device is presented in Figure 10-1. Sutureless catheter securement devices are another example of an engineering control. These devices

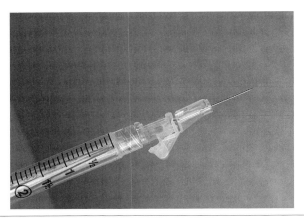

FIGURE 10-1 Safety needles help to reduce risk of a needlestick. *To activate the safety feature on this device, the plastic hinge is pushed with the fingertip after the injection, and the cover locks over the needle tip.*

are designed to reduce risk by stabilizing the intravenous insertion site to prevent restarting an IV unnecessarily. Eliminating the need for sutures to hold these devices in place further reduces the risk. (See Figure 10-2.)

Physicians prescribing oral rather than injectable medication, staff education, the use of standard precautions (including safe needle devices),

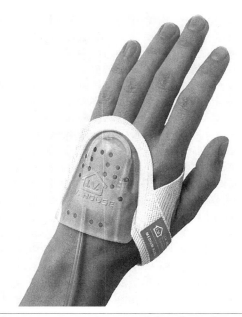

FIGURE 10-2 *Catheter securement devices stabilize the catheter at the insertion site. Well-secured sites may require less frequent site changes, saving time and reducing risk for both client and caregiver.*

elimination of needle recapping, and the use of sharps containers for proper disposal of sharps have demonstrated a reduction in needle-stick injuries. Other work practices include replacing sharps containers when three-quarters full; use of PPE such as goggles and face shields, gloves, masks, and gowns; eliminating the act of recapping needles; and placing sharps containers so that the syringe can go from the client directly into the sharps container.

Devices that have demonstrated the highest risk for BBP transmission are conventional butterfly needles, syringes used for blood collection, vacuum-tube phlebotomy needles, IV catheters, and blood-gas syringes. Glass capillary tubes and other glass items also pose greater risk because of the amount of blood to which the caregiver can potentially be exposed if injured.

Selection of Safe Sharps

The availability of safer sharps and medical devices has improved dramatically since the Needlestick Safety and Prevention Act was passed. Today, there are many safe device options to choose from. Although some institutions may have been reluctant to implement preventive strategies because of associated costs of the devices, use of such devices is required by law (with few exceptions).

Selecting Safe Sharps Disposal Containers

The design of sharps disposal containers is intended to minimize hazards associated with disposal and should not create additional hazards. Sharps containers must be red in color or labeled with the biohazard symbol. (See Figures 10-4 and 10-5.)

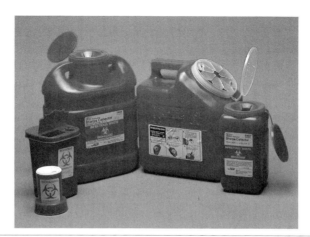

FIGURE 10-4 Examples of sharps disposal containers. *Sharps containers should be durble, closable, leak resistant on their sides and bottoms, either red in color or labeled with the biohazard symbol, and puncture resistant until final disposal.*

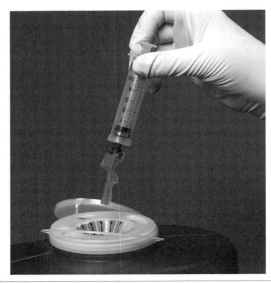

FIGURE 10-5 *Sharps containers should be emptied when they are no more than three-quarters full. Full containers can cause contaminated devices to become "hung-up" or to bounce back out of the container.*

OSHA Training Requirements

Training for prevention of BBP transmission is required initially at the time of job assignment and annually thereafter. OSHA requires employers to cover specific topics in an interactive environment where questions can be asked of the person conducting the training session. Required topics include the epidemiology and symptoms of bloodborne diseases and how they are transmitted, an explanation of the appropriate methods for recognizing tasks and other activities that may involve exposure to blood and OPIM and how exposure can be prevented, appropriate actions to take and persons to contact in an emergency involving blood or OPIM, exposure incident procedures, and method of medical follow-up.

MANAGEMENT OF BBP EXPOSURE INCIDENTS

Caregivers should follow facility policy for reporting and seeking treatment for BBP exposure incidents. Typical steps are summarized below and outlined in Table 10-1.

First Aid and Reporting

Clean the wound thoroughly with soap and water, and cover. Flush splashes to the nose, mouth, or skin with copious amounts of water. Irrigate eyes with

TABLE 10-1 Summary of Actions for a Potential Bloodborne Pathogen Exposure

1. Provide immediate care to the exposure site.
2. Determine risk associated with exposure.
3. Evaluate exposure source.
4. Evaluate and counsel the exposed person.
5. Give postexposure prophylaxis if indicated for exposures posing risk of disease.
6. Provide follow-up testing and counseling.

Source: Adapted from Appendix B, Guidelines for the Management of Occupational Exposures to HBV, HCB, and HIV and Recommendations for Postexposure Prophylaxis, Centers for Disease Control and Prevention, June, 2001.

clean water, saline, or sterile irrigants. Do not use bleach or other chemical disinfectant on the skin unless specifically designed for skin cleansing. Report the event to the supervisor.

The Importance of Seeking Immediate Medical Attention

The exposed caregiver should be evaluated promptly; the nature and severity of the exposure is also evaluated (type of body substance, route, device, volume) to ascertain appropriate treatment. Generally, drugs used to reduce or eliminate the likelihood of HIV transmission should be initiated as soon as possible, ideally within 2 hours. Although most exposures do not require prophylactic medications, in addition to the medical evaluation needed to assess the risk, counseling is needed to inform the caregiver of the nature of the risk, warning signs, and temporary lifestyle changes that may be needed to protect loved ones. Laboratory testing is performed on both exposed and source individuals when possible. This testing can be refused, but is recommended as it helps to guide the appropriate treatment. The testing provides caregiver baseline infection and immunity status and knowledge of source client infection status; both assist the medical provider in determining whether prophylactic medications are indicated.

Follow-up Testing

The caregivers' blood may be tested periodically over the next 6 months, depending on source client laboratory results and overall exposure risk assessment. It is well documented that transmission of these diseases most frequently occurs within 6 months of exposure.

PART 4

EMERGENCY MANAGEMENT AND SECURITY

CHAPTER

11

PREVENTING WORKPLACE VIOLENCE IN THE HEALTH CARE SETTING

INTRODUCTION

Workplace violence is any violent act directed toward a person who is at work or on duty. It can be inflicted on caregivers from internal (coworkers, clients) as well as external (robbers, intimate partners) sources.

A violent act can vary in severity from offensive words to murder. It includes but is not limited to abuse, threats, harassment, assaults, and muggings. *Abuse* is verbal or nonverbal mistreatment. A *threat* specifically involves an expression of intent to harm and can also be verbal, either written or spoken, or nonverbal, such as aggressive body language. *Harassment* can be physical, sexual, or emotional, and often takes the form of unwanted sexual advances or bullying. Harassment typically includes words or behaviors repeatedly directed at a particular person that annoy, alarm, or cause that person substantial emotional distress. *Assaults* are verbal or nonverbal attacks and may involve weapons. *Muggings* are assaults that are usually conducted with the intent to commit robbery.

Workplace violence may also include abuse through the improper use of power and control.

TYPES OF WORKPLACE VIOLENCE

Workplace violence incidents generally fall into four categories:

Type I, Criminal Intent

Type II, Client–Worker

Type III, Worker-on-Worker

Type IV, Personal Relationships

Type I, Criminal Intent

Workplace violence with criminal intent typically involves a perpetrator who does not have a legitimate business relationship with the employee or business and becomes violent in the process of committing a crime, often theft. A weapon is usually involved. Bystanders may be injured because of their proximity to the crime or their desire to help.

Type II, Client–Worker

A customer being served by the business or organization may become violent and injure or threaten a worker. This category of workplace violence is the type most commonly seen in health care settings.

Type III, Worker-on-Worker

Type III violence occurs when an employee, or former employee, is motivated to violence by unresolved personal or work-related conflicts. The most serious form of this type of violence is homicide. Although this usually involves an employee and supervisor/manager, coworkers can become injured or killed in the process.

Worker-on-worker violence also includes a much broader and more subtle form of violence, including harassment, bullying, verbal or emotional abuse, intimidation, unwanted sexual advances, veiled threats, misuse of authority and power, and other behaviors that create a stressful and anxiety-ridden workplace. Caregivers are often reluctant to report concerns to management. Management should deal with these types of situations in a confidential manner by protecting the name of the reporting employee.

Confrontation is difficult, but delivering a timely, professional but direct statement such as "Your behavior is offensive to me; please stop" can be very effective. In some cases the perpetrator may not realize that the behavior is offensive and will stop the behavior when confronted. This type of direct communication should never be attempted with threats of physical harm;

rather it may be appropriate only in less severe forms of abuse. Threats of violence should be reported immediately.

Type IV, Personal Relationships

Intimate partner violence (IPV) is physical, sexual, or psychological harm inflicted by one person over a less powerful person in an intimate relationship. IPV frequently spills over to the work environment.

Perpetrators of IPV may seek their victim in the workplace when restraining orders or other obstacles make locating their victim outside of work more difficult. Caregivers in all health care settings should stay alert for signs of impending IPV, report threats immediately, and be trained in extrication and self-protection strategies. **Extrication** involves removing oneself from the situation.

The Corporate Alliance to End Partner Violence (CAEPV) is a national organization focused on assisting employers with developing effective IPV violence-prevention strategies. A wide variety of workplace policy development and training materials are available on their Web site. Consult the text on which this guide is based, *Working Safely in Health Care, A Practical Guide*, for additional information on how to access information from this Web site.

Caregivers can be victims of IPV in their own relationships. Anyone suffering abuse from an intimate partner should be aware that help is available through local and national domestic violence prevention agencies.

All health care professionals should be trained to recognize the signs and symptoms of IPV and learn effective intervention strategies appropriate to the clinical setting. Victims of IPV feel a great deal of shame and humiliation about their situation. Myths about abuse persist in our culture and reinforce beliefs that the victim is free to leave the relationship at any time; victims stay with their abusers because they are afraid to leave. Victims of IPV are three times more likely to be killed or suffer severe injury on leaving the relationship.

Simply asking "Is someone you care about hurting you?" can be an effective method of asking about abuse. Help with creating a safety plan, finding a safe house (shelter), and securing financial assistance is available through local and national domestic violence prevention organizations. Obtain written information from local and national agencies in advance to have available to provide to abuse victims.

RISK FACTORS FOR WORKPLACE VIOLENCE

Risk factors can be grouped as societal, organizational, or environmental, and individual behaviors that are associated with an increased risk of illness or injury. Societal risk factors are often out of the direct control of the individual. However, organizational and individual risk factors, when identified, can be greatly reduced by implementing well-established and proven risk-reduction strategies.

Societal Risk Factors

Societal risk factors are intricately woven into the fabric of our community behaviors and norms. As violence continues, more and more agitated and frightened clients and family members are entering the health care system. Fear can cause normally rational individuals to lose the ability to cope, and, as they lose control, or **decompensate,** they may strike out verbally or physically. Individuals can help solve these problems by getting involved in local community efforts aimed at improving societal conditions.

Cost-containment strategies in the mental health setting have resulted in chronically and severely mentally ill individuals being released into mainstream society with little support. These individuals usually rely on medications to maintain their tenuous hold on reality—medications they may forget to take or cannot afford to purchase. As these individuals decompensate, some exhibit violent behaviors and enter the criminal justice system, in which medical treatment may be inappropriate or limited at best.

Organizational and Environmental Risk Factors

Managers who take potential threats of violence seriously and take appropriate violence-prevention measures reduce the risk for all in the organization. Caregivers can help by forming a multidisciplinary violence-prevention team to identify potential risks and make recommendations for improvement.

Extensive training is critical; emotions intensify during a threat situation and caregivers must rely on this training for the safety of all involved. Some organizations conduct routine drills to reinforce these important skills.

Individual Behaviors

Strong coping, communication, and stress-management skills help individuals effectively manage conflict. **Burnout,** a condition of extreme stress and exhaustion, can make a person more vulnerable to workplace violence. See additional information on stress management in Chapter 15.

Developing conflict-resolution skills can equip the caregiver to identify and manage conflict as it begins to emerge. Individuals can seek out formal training on communication skills and conflict resolution on their own if their employer does not offer it. Training resources on communication and conflict management may also be available at little or no cost through the local library, the local community education network, on the Internet, or through the employer's **Employee Assistance Program (EAP).** Although not all health care organizations have them, Employee Assistance Programs can be an excellent resource for information and help. An EAP is a benefit offered by some employers that provides employee access to basic mental health services. Some EAPs offer training, as well.

When entering into a difficult conflict-resolution discussion, avoid distraction; it is best for the caregiver to respect privacy and establish rules of engagement early. The caregiver should avoid starting discussions with how the other person should change behavior. Instead, using "I"-centered statements may effectively communicate the impact of the behavior and the expected consequences if behavior continues; for example, "I am offended by your comments, and I have documented them. I will be bringing this issue up at your care conference next week." This communication strategy is based on the principle that the caregiver is powerless to change, control, or be responsible for another individual's feelings, thoughts, or actions. It helps to keep the process objective and minimizes blaming dialog.

Open, honest, and timely communication is the basis for preventing conflict and for prompt resolution should conflict arise. Unresolved or ongoing individual or team conflict should be reported to management when repeated attempts to ask the perpetrator to stop the offending behavior have failed, when the threat of violence is escalating, or when authority is being misused.

Learning which communication techniques are most effective with a difficult client can take patience and creativity. Once a technique has been discovered, the caregiver should incorporate this method into the care plan for others to consider. Communicating behaviors deemed to be unacceptable, and reporting incidents or near misses, is very important to continuity of care, and to the safety of others on the unit.

PHASES OF VIOLENCE

An interaction or conflict with a client or coworker can escalate through the three phases of violence—baseline, preassault, and assault—in a matter of seconds, or it may take weeks or months. The alert caregiver can often detect warning signals and intervene. If the intervention is effective, the individual's baseline is restored; if not, the behavior may escalate. It is important for the caregiver to be aware of behaviors associated with each phase.

Baseline Phase

The term **baseline phase** is used to describe normal demeanor; the individual is demonstrating behavior deemed normal for that individual. Caregivers should learn about a client's normal or baseline mental and behavioral status prior to rendering care.

Preassault Phase

The **preassault phase** is characterized by an escalation of emotions and actions. The client begins to display threatening verbal and nonverbal cues as agitation increases. Verbal agitation may be evidenced by abusive remarks, loud, rapid speech, and profanity. Motor agitation may manifest as a subtle change in posture, clenching and unclenching of fists, pacing or fidgeting, gritted teeth, flushed face, rapid breathing, widened eyes, and flaring nostrils.

In some cases, especially in clients with a mental health disorder, a sudden change in level of consciousness, such as confusion and hallucinations, may signal impending violence. Impending violence may also manifest as a sudden change in outward appearance of emotion, or **affect.** The client may suddenly appear exhilarated or grandiose or, to the other extreme, suddenly display a calm affect when the client was previously agitated. Either extreme may be an indication that the client has made a decision to commit a violent act. Intoxication with any mind-altering substance can also be a warning signal.

Cues in coworkers can be identical to those described in the preassault phase in clients, but may not be recognized until escalation is well under way. Preassault behavior in a coworker may manifest as general job dissatisfaction and is often accompanied by emotional volatility. Most health care organizations have a policy for reporting and managing threatening behavior, but even if there is no policy, caregivers should report such behavior. Reporting should not reflect opinion; rather the caregiver should carefully and objectively document specific behaviors and record specific comments, including action taken.

Assault Phase

In the **assault phase** the individual loses control of both verbal and physical behavior, striking out at the person perceived as the cause of his or her anger or, in some cases, at the closest target. In this heightened emotional phase, attempts to verbally calm the individual will usually be ineffective and can actually intensify the reaction. Immediate reactions should be centered on extricating individuals from the immediate environment, isolating the violent individual, and activating the organization's emergency response system.

DE-ESCALATION TECHNIQUES

De-escalation refers to the ability to recognize a threat and to know when and how to attempt to defuse it. There are times when a potentially violent situation has already escalated when the caregiver enters the situation. Intervention should be in accordance with employer policy, and responses will differ depending on the severity of the situation. Good communication and conflict-resolution skills are essential in any potentially volatile situation. Regardless of how the caregiver may be feeling, every effort should be made to appear calm and to demonstrate compassion. A nonthreatening posture and body language should be maintained.

It is important for the caregiver to keep in mind that agitated individuals are unable to process complex information; verbal instructions should be simple, clear, and direct. Boundaries should be established with clear behavioral expectations; for example, "I can understand your anger, and I think we might be able to solve the problem if we can step into the hallway and talk."

Using **reflective communication** can be an effective method to check for understanding and maintain a nonthreatening dialog. Reflective communication involves restating client comments, and directing them back to the client. The caregiver should be especially aware of voice inflection and tone, and volume and rate of speech, as such communication characteristics can be misinterpreted. It is also best to avoid trying to have a conversation when the agitated client is shouting. Generally, it is recommended that the client be allowed to express grievances freely, with the caregiver responding selectively to clear up misconceptions and to acknowledge valid complaints. A comment such as "I know you must be tired of waiting" is an example of identifying and validating that the caregiver is aware of the situation and that client concerns will be addressed, while not reacting to the client's abusive statements. Silence can be used effectively; it provides an opportunity for the agitated client to clarify thoughts.

In addition to assuming a position between the client and the door to allow for quick exit if it is needed, the caregiver should maintain a distance of about 6 feet to avoid crowding an agitated individual. Rather than face the aggressive individual, it is recommended that the caregiver stand at a 90-degree angle to the client, with feet slightly apart. It will likely be perceived as less threatening if arms are relaxed at the side with palms facing forward. Direct eye contact can be intimidating. Table 11-1 lists examples of suggested actions when violence may be imminent.

TABLE 11-1   Suggested Actions When Violence May Be Imminent

R	**Remove.** Staff should leave the area and avoid the temptation for immediate intervention. A crisis is not the most appropriate time to develop a plan.
O	**Organize** staff to respond as a team to limit access to the area, and immediately notify security personnel, giving them the exact location of the disturbance.
A	**Assign.** Limit the number of caregivers handling the situation. Assign one staff member to deal with the client, another to control onlookers, and another to call for backup help and direct emergency responders to the scene.
D	**De-escalate.** Limit the number of staff in the room to as few as possible but have sufficient staff at hand should they be needed. Use de-escalation techniques appropriate to the situation.

Source: Adapted from DeReuter, H. (2004, July). *Best practices for safe patient handling and movement related to cognitively impaired/agitated patients.* Presented at the Healthcare Ergonomics Conference, Portland, OR.

Well-researched violence predictors form the basis of an individual violence risk assessment. The predictive characteristics include but are not limited to the following:

- Externalizes blame. Refuses to take responsibility for actions.

- Holds extremist opinions and attitudes.

- Has poor self-esteem. Needs to be right. Does not acknowledge limitations or need for help for personal problems.

- Has a history of involvement with alcohol or other drugs.

- Owns or is fascinated with weapons. May have had weapons training in the military.

- Has a history of poor work evaluations. Has trouble accepting constructive feedback. Holds grudges, especially against management or others in authority.

- Is fascinated with media violence or violent literature.

- Is usually a loner and is often withdrawn.

- Tests the limits of socially acceptable behavior.

- Has a history of failed relationships and a history of abuse.

It is important to note that these are general personality traits and should be considered in the context of the situation. Because of safety and legal considerations, a violence risk assessment should always be conducted with at least two members of the violence-response team in attendance, with backup security personnel readily available and documentation carefully and objectively recorded.

Violence Prevention Controls

An effective program will use a combination of engineering, administrative, and work-practice controls and personal protective equipment (PPE). Engineering controls for workplace violence focus on structural improvements such as redesign of waiting and triage areas, improved lighting in dark corridors and parking areas, and installation of metal detectors, panic buttons, and alarm systems in high-risk areas.

Administrative and work-practice controls consist of policies and procedures, including reporting procedures, training, and other prevention interventions related to manager and employee work practices. Ongoing caregiver training is important. Training content should include, but is not limited to:

- Review of written policy and location of policy for future reference

- Risk factors for violence and high-risk client-care areas

- Communication and conflict-resolution strategies
- Behavioral and emotional warning signs of escalating violence
- Violence de-escalation strategies
- Self-protection and extrication strategies
- When and how to call for help
- Incident documentation and auditing procedures
- Policy and procedure for reporting coworker or supervisor violence
- Postincident debriefing services, including referral to professional services

Additional administrative controls may include:

- Enforcing visitor hours and procedures and establishing a list of restricted visitors for clients with a history of violence or gang activity
- Limiting information released about hospitalized victims of violence
- Control of client movement throughout the facility
- Controlled public access to areas other than waiting rooms
- Adequate staffing levels to prevent caregivers from working alone in high-risk or isolated areas
- Communication system to identify clients with potentially violent tendencies or a history of violent behavior
- Security escorts to parking facilities
- Work plan for field staff members to keep a designated contact person informed about their whereabouts throughout the day

There are few examples in which PPE is effective in *preventing* a workplace violence incident, but judicious use of PPE may reduce the risk of an adverse outcome in certain circumstances. Using PPE such as surgical masks and safety eyewear for clients who spit can prevent exposure incidents that may result from workplace violence incidents. Each client-care situation should be evaluated carefully to determine whether PPE is an appropriate control.

Preventing Workplace Violence in the Home-Care Environment

Before entering any unfamiliar client-care environment, the caregiver should assess the environment for potential violence indicators or other safety or health hazards. It is prudent to observe the surrounding environment on the initial visit, observing restaurants, police stations, and other safe environments that may be used as a refuge if needed. Upon entry, the caregiver should assume a position between the client and the door to allow for a quick and direct exit if needed.

Caregivers should be alert to people sitting in parked cars and walk briskly, making direct eye contact with the people around them. Walking against the flow of traffic allows the caregiver to observe approaching vehicles. Care should be taken to check the outside of the vehicle as well as the front and backseats before getting into the car and to lock car doors immediately. Home environments present unique challenges, but the risk of violence can be significantly decreased by using these safe work practices.

Consult the text on which this guide is based, *Working Safely in Health Care, A Practical Guide*, for additional information on personal safety when caring for a client in his or her home.

Postincident Response

Postincident response refers to those activities conducted following the incident to help the organization and caregivers return to a normal state. This includes debriefing the involved caregivers, collecting and reviewing relevant documentation, and reporting to external law enforcement or other local authorities. Postincident stress debriefing for caregivers (and psychological assistance, if indicated) is important, regardless of the severity of the violence.

It is essential that the incident be recorded objectively. Incident documentation should be used in an after-action review to critique event response to explore what went well and what could be improved in an effort to identify programming gaps or additional training needs. Documentation may include:

- Name of victim or potential victims
- Location, date, and time the incident occurred
- Events immediately prior and leading up to the incident
- The specific language of the threat
- Physical conduct that would substantiate an intention to follow through on the threat
- How the threat-maker appeared, physically and emotionally
- Names of other individuals who were directly involved and any actions they took

- Incident outcome, including transport location of any individuals involved in the event
- Extent of any injuries, and evaluation methods
- Names and contact numbers of witnesses
- Disposition of the perpetrator after the incident
- List of community emergency services that may have been activated

CHAPTER

12

EMERGENCY MANAGEMENT AND TERRORISM

EMERGENCY MANAGEMENT

Emergency management is the organization and management of resources and responsibilities to handle all aspects of emergencies and disasters. Elements of emergency management are mitigation, preparedness, response, and recovery. **Mitigation** includes measures taken to reduce the probability of an event, or to reduce the severity, loss, or consequences, either prior to or following a disaster or catastrophe. **Preparedness** encompasses the plans and strategies developed prior to an emergency that are used to improve and support mitigation, response, and recovery efforts in the event of a disaster or catastrophic event. **Response,** in the context of this chapter, includes actions taken to save lives and prevent further damage in a disaster or emergency. Response is putting preparedness plans into action. **Recovery** is the cleanup stage, usually composed of activities and programs designed to return conditions to a level so that operations can resume. The four phases of emergency management are summarized in Figure 12-1.

Mitigation

Mitigation includes measures taken to reduce the probability of an incident, or to reduce the severity, loss, or consequences if an incident occurs. The

Mitigation: 1) Hazard identification 2) Hazard elimination and control 3) Training and education	Preparedness: 1) Hazard vulnerability analysis 2) Identification of resources 3) Establishment of guidelines, protocols, and standards
Response: 1) Immediate actions to save lives, protect property, and meet basic human needs 2) Security 3) Public health measures	Recovery: Restoration of social, economic, environmental, and governmental services to facilitate return to pre-disaster levels

FIGURE 12-1 The four phases of emergency management.

goal is to save lives and reduce property damage. Mitigation efforts have the most impact if carried out prior to an incident.

Whatever the type of disaster, these are the key steps to the mitigation process.

Hazard Identification

Hazard identification includes listing all emergencies that could impact the home, facility, or community, including those identified by the local emergency management office. These will vary depending on historical, geographical, and technological factors, human error, and the actual physical characteristics of the building and the community.

Hazard Elimination and Control

Hazard elimination and control is the process of preventing or reducing the potential for an identified hazard to impact your facility or community.

Training and Education

A prepared and knowledgeable workforce is essential in reducing the potential impact of any emergency. The employer should repeat training frequently and invite coordination with outside agencies at local, county, state, and federal levels when practical. Each caregiver's responsibility is to actively participate in training sessions and drills and apply what has been learned both at work and at home.

Preparedness

Preparedness takes the form of plans or procedures designed to save lives and to minimize damage to property when a disaster or emergency occurs. Planning, training, and disaster drills are essential elements of preparedness.

These activities ensure that when a disaster strikes, the individuals involved will know what actions are necessary to provide the best response possible. Having a disaster plan is one of the strongest predictors of the ability to recover from a disaster.

At a personal level, preparedness involves developing a family emergency plan. Preparedness is a continuous process that includes the hazard vulnerability analysis.

Hazard Vulnerability Analysis

The **hazard vulnerability analysis** is an estimate of the probability and potential impact of each emergency that might affect your home, community, or region. The analysis is used to assess hazards and produce a rating of the likelihood of such an occurrence, the potential severity, and the level of preparedness. The resulting score reflects overall vulnerability. An excerpt of a hazard vulnerability analysis is provided in Figure 12-2.

Response

Response is defined as the actions taken to save lives and prevent further damage in a disaster or emergency. Response is putting preparedness plans into action. Depending on the type of emergency or disaster, response could include damage assessment, search and rescue, evacuation, firefighting, and sheltering and treating victims, or it could include increased security, public health monitoring, testing of potentially exposed populations, and immunizations.

Type of Emergency	Probability		Human Impact	Property Impact	Business Impact	Internal Resources	External Resources	Total
	High Low ←——→ 5 1		High Impact ←———————— 5		Low Impact 1	Weak Resources ←———— 5	Strong Resources ——→ 1	
Earthquake	4		5	5	5	2	3	**24**
Terrorist Attack	2		5	4	3	1	2	**17**
Fire	3		4	4	3	4	4	**22**

FIGURE 12-2 Excerpt from a hazard vulnerability analysis for a hospital on the west coast of the United States. *This example evaluates three potential hazards for probability of occurrence; the potential impact on humans, property, and business; and the resources currently in place to manage each event. Each is rated on a scale of 1 to 5. The analysis shows that the lowest hazard is the terrorist attack, with total points of 17. The highest is the earthquake, with a total of 23 points; perhaps this hospital is located on a major fault. The fire hazard risk is 22; perhaps this hospital is in a forested, fire-prone area. A similar system can be used to evaluate personal preparedness.*

Recovery

Recovery is defined as the actions taken to return the community to normal following a disaster. On a personal level, recovery will include those actions taken to ensure personal health and safety and the initiation of steps necessary to resume normal daily life, such as arranging for a safe and secure location for important documents that will be needed following a disaster.

Recovery also means taking care of physical and mental health concerns. Use of support groups is one method; one of the best ways to cope with the stress of a disaster is to try to return to normal daily activities as soon as possible.

Depending on the type of disaster, awareness of safety hazards in and around the health care facility and the caregiver's home and neighborhood will be critical to recovery. On a broader level, recovery includes the development, coordination, and execution of service- and site-restoration plans. It also involves the restoration of personal and governmental operations and services. An important part of the recovery process should include the evaluation of the incident to identify lessons learned and the initiation of measures to minimize the effects of future incidents.

People often feel that preparing for and responding to the event are the most important aspects, yet if a person is unable to return to normal operating conditions at home or at work, the plan has not been effective. The ability to recover defines the long-term impact and severity of the disaster.

INCIDENT COMMAND SYSTEM

An **incident command system** is an organizational arrangement using a chain of command in which individuals use a standardized reporting structure to deal with small and large incidents. The **incident commander** is responsible for overseeing the development and implementation of the emergency plan.

The mission of the incident command is to define the mission and make sure it is completed using the four structural elements summarized in Figure 12-3. The incident command plan changes, and is dependent on the emergency or disaster that has occurred. Success of this system is dependent on continuous communication among the four elements, and this helps achieve the best disaster response possible. The incident command system is summarized in Figure 12-3.

Hospital Incident Command System

A key resource for health care disaster readiness is the **hospital incident command system (HICS).** It is becoming the standard for health care

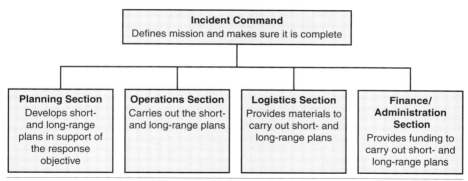

FIGURE 12-3 A typical incident command structure.

disaster response in a hospital setting. It uses a logical management structure, defined responsibilities, clear reporting channels, and a common language to help unify the hospital response with community, state, and federal emergency response efforts.

TERRORISM

Terrorism-related acts and events have become more frequent and widely reported in the media. Defining terrorism can assist the caregiver to better understand this phenomenon and thus be better prepared to deal with the possibility of an attack.

The **Department of Homeland Security** is the agency within the U.S. government charged primarily with securing the nation and protecting citizens from terrorist threats. The Homeland Security Act of 2002 defines **terrorism** as activity that involves an act dangerous to human life or potentially destructive of critical infrastructure or key resources *and is intended to intimidate or coerce the civilian population or influence a government by mass destruction, assassination, or kidnapping* in violation of the criminal laws of the United States. Terrorist objectives may be political, religious, or ideological. Terrorism is a specific kind of violence.

Managing Terrorism

Managing terrorism includes both antiterrorism and counterterrorism activities. **Antiterrorism** refers to defensive measures used to reduce the vulnerability of people and property to terrorist acts, while **counterterrorism** includes offensive measures taken to prevent, deter, and respond to terrorism. Thus, antiterrorism is an element of hazard mitigation, while counterterrorism falls within the scope of preparedness, response, and recovery.

Types of Terrorism

Terrorist acts can take many forms. **Intellectual terrorism,** which is the use of propaganda or other biased messages to encourage religious, cultural, or political support for the terrorists, may be one of the most dangerous types of terrorism. These messages may not be true or may not paint a full picture of the facts. Using discrimination, prejudice, hatred, exclusion, slander, mockery, and humiliation are just a few ways intellectual terrorism is used.

Weapons of Mass Destruction

Most recently, certain forms of terrorism described as **weapons of mass destruction (WMD)** have received particular attention. WMD include **chemical** and **biological agents, explosive devices, radiological materials,** and **nuclear weapons,** often described by the acronym **CBERN,** used to create fear, injury, and death on a large (mass) scale. These methods are primarily associated with terrorist organizations and rogue governments and are described in the following paragraphs.

Chemical Terrorism

Chemical agents are chemical hazards used in terrorism. They may include poisonous vapors, aerosols, liquids, and solids that have toxic effects on people, animals, or plants. They may be released by bombs or sprayed from aircraft, boats, and vehicles. They can be used as a liquid to create a hazard to people and the environment. Some chemical agents may be odorless and tasteless. They can have an immediate effect (a few seconds to a few minutes) or a delayed effect (2 to 48 hours). Although potentially lethal, chemical agents are difficult to deliver in lethal concentrations. Outdoors, the agents often dissipate rapidly. Chemical agents also are difficult to produce.

A chemical attack could come without warning. Signs of a chemical release include people having difficulty breathing, experiencing eye irritation, losing coordination, becoming nauseated, or having a burning sensation in the nose, throat, and lungs. Also, the presence of many dead insects or birds may indicate release of a chemical agent.

Biological Terrorism

Biological agents are biological and infectious hazards that can kill or incapacitate people, livestock, and crops. The three basic groups of biological agents that would likely be used as weapons are pathogens such as bacteria (e.g., anthrax or cholera) and viruses (e.g., smallpox or pneumonic plague), and **toxins** (i.e., poisonous substances) obtained from certain organisms and plants.

Most biological agents are difficult to grow and maintain. Biological agents may be dispersed by spraying them into the air, by infecting animals that carry the disease to humans, and by contaminating food and water.

The caregiver is very likely to be in a position to detect a bioterrorist attack. To prepare for this possibility, it is important for the caregiver to maintain an index of suspicion and to report such unusual presentations in an otherwise healthy population. Conditions seen in clusters or unusually high numbers within a short period of time may yield important clues. Acute onset of unusual symptoms (e.g., respiratory distress, severe diarrhea and dehydration, unexplained rash with fever, change in mental status) in a younger (<50 years) population, in the "wrong" season, and with no history of foreign travel should arouse suspicion.

In these situations it is very important for the caregiver to use appropriate isolation precautions (see Chapter 9) to prevent pathogen transmission. Clients with a cough should be asked to wear a surgical mask and be kept isolated if possible. Standard precautions, including hand hygiene, must be meticulously observed.

Any suspicion of a biological event should be immediately reported to proper authorities (usually the local public health department). Following notification, the public health department will arrange for specialized laboratory testing and provide guidelines for treatment and prompt immunization of the general population, if indicated. They will also begin a public health investigation and activate local, state, and federal emergency response systems.

Explosive Devices in Terrorism

Terrorists frequently use explosive devices in terrorism. These include bombs, rockets and grenades (stolen or illegally purchased), or explosives made from materials like dynamite. In addition, devices made from chemicals from agriculture and industries have been used by terrorists. The materials needed to construct an explosive device are easy to obtain. Explosive devices are highly portable, using vehicles and humans as a means of transport. They are easily detonated from remote locations or by suicide bombers.

Radiological Materials in Terrorism

Terrorists use radiological (radioactive) materials in terrorist activities, often in devices constructed by combining an explosive agent like dynamite with radioactive materials that may have been stolen from a hospital or local industry. The initial explosion kills or injures those closest to the bomb, while the tiny particles of radioactive material remain to contaminate survivors and emergency responders. These devices are called **radiological distribution devices (RDD),** or "dirty nukes" or "dirty bombs"; they appeal to terrorists because they require limited technical knowledge to build and deploy.

The primary purpose of terrorist use of an RDD is to cause psychological fear and economic disruption. An RDD may cause injuries and fatalities from the conventional explosive exposure or from exposure to radioactive materials contained in it. Health effects related to the radiological exposure will depend on the type of radiation involved, the extent and nature (dose) of the exposure, and the individual characteristics of the exposed individuals. External irradiation is not a medical emergency. Medical treatment is necessary, but health effects from the radiation exposure may not manifest for days to weeks.

To **shelter-in-place** provides immediate protection for people in the event of a disaster with airborne contamination such as would be produced by an RDD. Sheltering-in-place involves closing and locking all exterior doors and windows and retreating to an interior room (preferably with few windows) and staying there until public safety personnel advise that it is safe to go outdoors. Duct tape and plastic sheeting heavier than food wrap should be used to seal all cracks around doors, windows, and vents into the room.

If sheltering-in-place and evacuation are completed promptly, the number of deaths and injuries from an RDD might not be substantially greater than from a conventional bomb explosion. The size of the affected area and the level of destruction caused by an RDD depend on the sophistication and size of the conventional bomb, the type of radioactive material used, the quality and quantity of the radioactive material, and the local weather conditions, especially wind and precipitation. The area affected could be placed off-limits to the public for several months during cleanup efforts.

The most important thing for the caregiver to keep in mind in this situation is that promptly donning the appropriate personal protective equipment (PPE) and beginning client **decontamination** (removing contaminated clothing and washing the client with soap and water) is essential to expedite care for the injured and to minimize further radiation exposure to the injured and to those providing care. This is best accomplished by setting up a triage area outside the hospital. **Triage** is a process used to determine the need for and priority of care. The client is triaged and decontaminated and sent for treatment for injuries according to the facility's triage protocol. Staff dealing with radiation exposure victims must use protective clothing (gowns, caps, boots, masks, and two pairs of gloves). Clients' clothing must be removed and stored in properly labeled bags. Access to the decontamination area must be controlled at all times. Attention to these four principles will help guide how decontamination areas are set up, staffed, and controlled to minimize exposure:

- Time: The shorter the time in a radiation area, the less the exposure.

- Distance: The farther away one is from the source of the radiation, the less the exposure.

- Shielding: Although not always practical in emergency situations, shielding offered by barriers can reduce radiation exposure.

- Quantity: Being aware of the amount of radiation involved and limiting the amount when possible can reduce radiation exposure.

Nuclear Weapons in Terrorism

Nuclear devices may be small or large. All nuclear devices cause deadly effects when exploded, including blinding light, intense heat (thermal radiation), initial nuclear radiation, blast, and fires ignited by the heat pulse, as well as secondary fires. Injuries occur from the initial blast and from flying debris. For caregivers, the same principles apply as outlined in the section above, but the extent of possible exposure and injury will be greater. The probability of sheltering-in-place followed by evacuation is likely.

Homeland Security Advisory System

The Department of Homeland Security Advisory System was devised to provide a national framework and a comprehensive means to disseminate information regarding the risk of terrorist acts. This system provides warnings in the form of graduated "threat levels" that increase as the risk of the threat increases. (See Figure 12-4.)

Emergency Response Safety Considerations

How the emergency plan is used will depend on the situation. The caregiver location when the emergency occurs will affect how the plan is implemented. Communication is essential. There may be times when to shelter-in-place is the best and the safest option available.

An evacuation plan is developed for those times when the best option is to get as far away from the situation as possible. Clients will continue to need care, and injuries suffered during the emergency may complicate the situation. The evacuation plan should have more than one location option for alternative care for clients, and it is essential that records be kept of where each client was sent. The caregiver should know the process for transporting clients to a safe area. The situation can change rapidly, and those changes can result in unexpected decisions that may affect short- or long-range plans. Guidelines published by the **Federal Emergency Management Agency (FEMA)** are provided in Table 12-3. FEMA is the primary agency within the U.S. government with the mission to help prepare the nation for all hazards and effectively manage federal response and recovery efforts following any national incident.

Communication between individuals and organizations is considered one of the more important factors when dealing with an emergency. If the conventional communication lines are broken, alternative communication plans should be in place, such as using a "runner" to go between different areas with information.

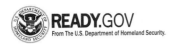

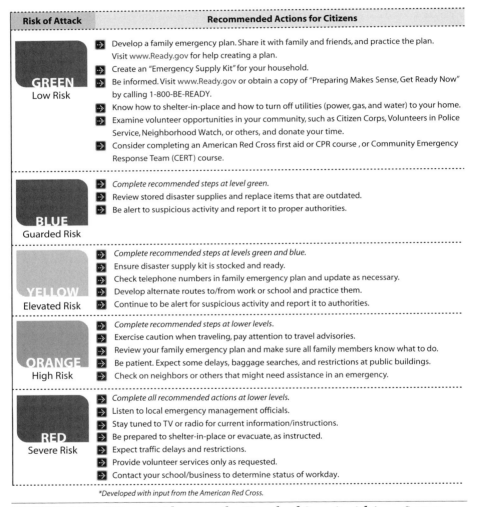

Citizen Guidance on the Homeland Security Advisory System

Risk of Attack	Recommended Actions for Citizens
GREEN Low Risk	Develop a family emergency plan. Share it with family and friends, and practice the plan. Visit www.Ready.gov for help creating a plan. Create an "Emergency Supply Kit" for your household. Be informed. Visit www.Ready.gov or obtain a copy of "Preparing Makes Sense, Get Ready Now" by calling 1-800-BE-READY. Know how to shelter-in-place and how to turn off utilities (power, gas, and water) to your home. Examine volunteer opportunities in your community, such as Citizen Corps, Volunteers in Police Service, Neighborhood Watch, or others, and donate your time. Consider completing an American Red Cross first aid or CPR course, or Community Emergency Response Team (CERT) course.
BLUE Guarded Risk	*Complete recommended steps at level green.* Review stored disaster supplies and replace items that are outdated. Be alert to suspicious activity and report it to proper authorities.
YELLOW Elevated Risk	*Complete recommended steps at levels green and blue.* Ensure disaster supply kit is stocked and ready. Check telephone numbers in family emergency plan and update as necessary. Develop alternate routes to/from work or school and practice them. Continue to be alert for suspicious activity and report it to authorities.
ORANGE High Risk	*Complete recommended steps at lower levels.* Exercise caution when traveling, pay attention to travel advisories. Review your family emergency plan and make sure all family members know what to do. Be patient. Expect some delays, baggage searches, and restrictions at public buildings. Check on neighbors or others that might need assistance in an emergency.
RED Severe Risk	*Complete all recommended actions at lower levels.* Listen to local emergency management officials. Stay tuned to TV or radio for current information/instructions. Be prepared to shelter-in-place or evacuate, as instructed. Expect traffic delays and restrictions. Provide volunteer services only as requested. Contact your school/business to determine status of workday.

Developed with input from the American Red Cross.

FIGURE 12-4 Citizen Guidance on the Homeland Security Advisory System.

The caregiver has the responsibility to take appropriate action in emergencies and disasters. Responding to an emergency is as important to quality client care as taking and interpreting vital signs, and may be even more important.

TABLE 12-3   The Federal Emergency Management Agency (FEMA)

FEMA has published the following general guidelines:

- Be aware of surroundings.
- Move or leave if things just do not feel right.
- Take precautions and be prepared when traveling for any unusual behaviors and/or suspicious items. Report these as soon as possible to authorities.
- Familiarize oneself with the location of emergency exits.
- Be prepared to do without services that are normally available, such as electricity, telephone, gas, and automated teller machines (ATMs).
- Have emergency kits available with flashlights, battery-operated radios, batteries, first-aid kits, and other items of necessity.

FIRE PREVENTION AND LIFE SAFETY

The caregiver role in fire prevention and life safety will vary based on the health care setting, but basic principles are unchanged. Fire prevention and life safety requires a team approach, and caregiver participation and cooperation is essential.

Mitigation activities include keeping hallways clear, prohibiting heat-producing devices such as space heaters in client-care areas, and inspecting medical equipment regularly. Preparedness activities include participating in fire drills and attending regular fire response training. It is important that the caregiver participate in these activities; clients expect caregivers to respond appropriately to a fire, and client and caregiver safety depends on a prompt and appropriate response. Responding to a fire emergency involves much more than simply moving a client from the fire area. The caregiver should be thoroughly familiar with facility policy related to appropriate fire response. Facility-specific training should address the caregiver role in detail. The acronym RACE (remove, activate, close, and extinguish) is widely used in health care to assist caregivers to remember the basic fire response steps. (See Table 12-4.)

TABLE 12-4   RACE

If you discover a fire, see flame or smoke, follow the RACE procedures:

R = Remove all persons in immediate danger to safe areas.

A = Activate the fire alarm AND call or direct someone to call 911.

C = Close doors to prevent the spread of smoke and fire.

E = Extinguish the fire if it is safe to do so.

Appropriate fire response includes knowledge of when evacuation is appropriate and how it is to be accomplished. The caregiver must know where clients are to be taken in the event of an evacuation and the procedures used to transport them, especially when safe areas are on lower floors and the elevators cannot be used. These procedures must be practiced regularly to ensure proficiency. Again, much of this information will be facility specific, and caregivers should seek opportunities to participate in fire drills and fire response training to become familiar with procedures in their facilities.

Evacuation generally falls into four main categories. Zone evacuation involves moving clients and personnel away from the immediate danger to an area within the same fire zone or fire compartment. This usually involves a small event and movement of a few clients. Caregivers should be familiar with fire zone boundaries in their work areas. Horizontal evacuation involves movement of clients to a predetermined evacuation area on the same floor (horizontally). This is the most common form of evacuation and is typically the type of evacuation practiced during routine fire drills. Floor (or vertical) evacuation requires movement of clients and personnel to another floor, usually to a floor below the fire event. It is used when horizontal evacuation is not sufficient and the floors below are safe areas. External evacuation to a predetermined assembly area can be a difficult and dangerous task in health care. It is typically ordered only in the event of a serious emergency. Some facilities require that external evacuation occur only at the direction of hospital administration or safety personnel or public safety personnel in charge at the scene.

Fire response includes knowledge of fire extinguisher locations, when and what type of extinguisher is appropriate, and how the extinguisher is used. Policies related to use of fire extinguishers are facility specific, but the acronym PASS (which stands for pull, aim, squeeze, and sweep) is commonly used to reinforce basic principles related to fire extinguisher use. (See Table 12-5.)

Fire response involves much more than using a fire extinguisher or moving clients, and maintaining ongoing caregiver proficiency is critical. Because facilities differ, fire planning and response differs. Caregivers should become familiar with all aspects of fire prevention and life safety in their facility—before a fire occurs.

TABLE 12-5 PASS

To remember the principles of fire extinguisher use, think of PASS:

P = Pull the locking pin

A = Aim the end of the hose at the base of the fire

S = Squeeze the handle

S = Sweep slowly from side to side

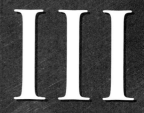

Section III

Wellness Challenges in Health care

CHAPTER

13

PERSONAL WELLNESS

INTRODUCTION

The body is designed to eliminate toxins and to withstand physical stress—within limits. These limits vary from individual to individual, but minimizing potentially hazardous exposures in the home and taking steps toward optimal health may help to reduce overall risk for injury or illness in the event of a hazardous exposure. Wellness is the result of wise lifestyle choices—good physical and mental health maintained by proper diet, exercise, and healthy self-care habits.

COMMON HAZARDS IN THE HOME ENVIRONMENT

The caregiver may encounter hazards in his or her home environment and leisure activities as well as in the workplace. The principles of hazard identification, elimination, and control can reduce overall risk at home just as in the work environment.

Indoor air quality concerns may also cause problems in the home. Exposure to the same substance at work and at home may increase the exposure dose.

Indoor Air Quality in the Home

Indoor air pollution in the home can come from a variety of sources, including:

* Environmental tobacco smoke

* Wood-burning stoves and gas ranges

* Building materials

* Asbestos

Household Products

Product warning labels on common household products may be inadequate. Material safety data sheets (MSDSs) are available from manufacturers on request for many of these products.

Lawn-Care Products

Pesticides and lawn-care products are potentially hazardous, especially to children. Pesticide exposure can occur through skin contact, inhalation, or ingestion. Proper use and storage of household pesticides and proper cleaning of food, especially raw fruits and vegetables, can help protect consumers.

Lead

Although lead was banned from paint for home use in 1972, millions of homes, particularly those built before 1950, may contain high amounts of lead in paint that is peeling and accessible for ingestion by children. Lead exposure also occurs through drinking water, especially in homes that have lead-soldered pipes, and through hobbies involving lead.

Recreational Health Hazards

Fishing and swimming in contaminated beaches, lakes, and streams can expose participants to hazardous chemicals and pathogens in polluted waters. Wooden playground structures that have not been sealed may allow children to have skin contact with potentially hazardous wood preservatives. Materials used in arts and crafts involve potentially hazardous silica, talc, solvents, and heavy metals such as lead and cadmium.

Water Supply

Public water supplies and private wells can be a source of hazardous chemical exposure, such as industrial solvents, heavy metals, pesticides, and fertilizers. Most municipalities have water quality results posted on Web sites available for public viewing.

Soil Contamination

Ingestion of contaminated soil poses a risk of adverse health effects, especially to children. Lead, dioxin, and certain pesticides may be found in soil. Other chemicals may be found in soil near existing or abandoned industrial sites.

MAINTAINING OPTIMAL HEALTH

Maintaining a high level of fitness and good nutrition will help to keep the body functioning at its best. Highlights of Centers for Disease Control and Prevention (CDC) recommendations related to fitness and nutrition are summarized below.

Understanding the Body's Energy Needs

Weight loss requires that more calories be burned than ingested. The Body Mass Index table presented in Table 4-1 in Chapter 4 can assist in assessing whether weight loss is needed. To maintain a healthy weight, calories burned must be in balance with calories ingested.

Calories versus Good Nutrition

The entire amount of calories needed in a day could be used up on a few high-calorie foods, but it is unlikely that the body would receive the full range of vitamins and nutrients needed for good health. The U.S. Department of Agriculture has published the Food Guide Pyramid to assist in helping individuals get adequate nutrition and maintain the energy balance. (See Figure 13-1.)

Balancing Food Intake and Physical Activity

Physical activity at moderate intensity for at least 30 minutes most days of the week is recommended. Increasing the intensity or the amount of time engaged in physical activity can have even greater health benefits and may be needed to control body weight. About 60 minutes a day may be needed to prevent weight gain. Table 13-1, adapted from the U.S. Department of Health and Human Services and U.S. Department of Agriculture's *Dietary Guidelines for Americans 2005*, provides examples of calorie expenditures per hour for various moderate and vigorous activities, based on a 154-pound individual. Calories burned per hour will be higher for persons who weigh more than 154 pounds and lower for persons who weigh less.

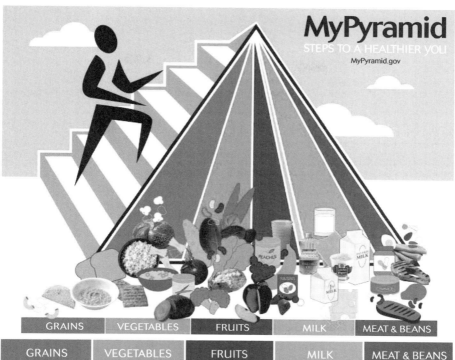

GRAINS Make half your grains whole	VEGETABLES Vary your veggies	FRUITS Focus on fruits	MILK Get your calcium-rich foods	MEAT & BEANS Go lean with protein
Eat at least 3 oz. of whole-grain cereals, breads, crackers, rice, or pasta every day 1 oz. is about 1 slice of bread, about 1 cup of breakfast cereal, or ½ cup of cooked rice, cereal, or pasta	Eat more dark-green veggies like broccoli, spinach, and other dark leafy greens Eat more orange vegetables like carrots and sweet potatoes Eat more dry beans and peas like pinto beans, kidney beans, and lentils	Eat a variety of fruit Choose fresh, frozen, canned, or dried fruit Go easy on fruit juices	Go low-fat or fat-free when you choose milk, yogurt, and other milk products If you don't or can't consume milk, choose lactose-free products or other calcium sources such as fortified foods and beverages	Choose low-fat or lean meats and poultry Bake it, broil it, or grill it Vary your protein routine — choose more fish, beans, peas, nuts, and seeds

For a 2,000-calorie diet, you need the amounts below from each food group. To find the amounts that are right for you, go to MyPyramid.gov.

Eat 6 oz. every day	Eat 2½ cups every day	Eat 2 cups every day	Get 3 cups every day; for kids aged 2 to 8, it's 2	Eat 5½ oz. every day

Find your balance between food and physical activity
- Be sure to stay within your daily calorie needs.
- Be physically active for at least 30 minutes most days of the week.
- About 60 minutes a day of physical activity may be needed to prevent weight gain.
- For sustaining weight loss, at least 60 to 90 minutes a day of physical activity may be required.
- Children and teenagers should be physically active for 60 minutes every day, or most days.

Know the limits on fats, sugars, and salt (sodium)
- Make most of your fat sources from fish, nuts, and vegetable oils.
- Limit solid fats like butter, margarine, shortening, and lard, as well as foods that contain these.
- Check the Nutrition Facts label to keep saturated fats, trans fats, and sodium low.
- Choose food and beverages low in added sugars. Added sugars contribute calories with few, if any, nutrients.

MyPyramid.gov
STEPS TO A HEALTHIER YOU

U.S. Department of Agriculture
Center for Nutrition Policy and Promotion
April 2005
CNPP-15

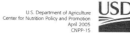

FIGURE 13-1 The U.S. Department of Agriculture's MyPyramid is a simple guide to a healthy lifestyle.

TABLE 13-1 Examples of Calorie Expenditures per Hour

Moderate Physical Activity	Approximate Calories/Hr for a 154-Pound Person
Hiking	370
Light gardening or yard work	330
Dancing	330
Golfing (walking and carrying clubs)	330
Bicycling <10 mph	290
Walking 3.5 mph	280
Weight lifting (general light workout)	220
Stretching	180
Vigorous Physical Activity	**Approximate Calories/Hr for a 154-Pound Person**
Running/jogging 5 mph	590
Bicycling >10 mph	590
Swimming (slow freestyle laps)	510
Aerobics	480
Walking 4.5 mph	460
Heavy yard work (chopping wood)	440
Weight lifting (vigorous effort)	440
Basketball (vigorous)	440

Source: Adapted from Dietary Guidelines for Americans 2005.

Emotional Wellness

Emotional wellness is the ability to cope with stress and maintain satisfying relationships. It includes the desire to learn, problem solve, and be creative. It is developing a sense of humor and an optimistic attitude. Emotional wellness is the ability to embrace normal emotions and not be immobilized by them. Emotional wellness is setting boundaries. Emotional wellness is also sensitivity to individual tolerance and knowing when additional support or professional help is needed.

Spiritual Wellness

Spiritual wellness is finding purpose and developing beliefs and values that give the caregiver direction in life. Spiritual wellness helps build a capacity to care for others. Spiritual health is individualized and includes respecting the beliefs of others.

Seeking Preventive Medical Care

Preventing disease is an important aspect of wellness. Individual risk factors determine the frequency of certain screenings and physical examinations. Using preventive medical services may avert the development of serious and disabling diseases and conditions.

Healthy Self-Care

Attentiveness to signs and symptoms and responding accordingly is another important aspect of wellness. Activities such as resting, taking a vacation, or spending time with a good book are important to wellness. It is also important to seek medical attention promptly when appropriate.

CHAPTER

14

SURVIVING SHIFT WORK SAFELY

THE NATURE OF SHIFT WORK

The American workweek has evolved into a medley of shifts, including day shift, evening shift, night shift, extended shift, split shift, rotating shift, and flextime. The health care setting providing 24-hour care will typically use two 12-hour shifts or three 8-hour shifts to staff the direct client-care departments. Other departments provide support to client care and may cover their services with one or more 8-hour shifts. The start time of work, consecutive workdays before a day off, and scheduling of weekends vary by facility and staffing model.

An **extended shift** is a shift lasting more than 8 hours. **Rotating shifts** are schedules involving a combination of day, night, and evening shifts, typically on a fixed schedule—for example, changing every 2 weeks. Rotating shifts are often used to provide equitable scheduling by providing a system in which all caregivers rotate through the less popular shifts. **Flextime** is a work arrangement mutually determined between the supervisor and caregiver that meets the needs of the work unit while providing additional flexibility for the caregiver. Not all health care settings are able to offer flextime. **On-call** workers typically carry pagers and are scheduled to be available for a certain period of time. The caregiver does not report to work during that time unless called, but if called, must report within a specified timeframe.

Caregivers often receive additional pay for working unpopular shifts and taking on-call time, but the unusual and sometimes unpredictable schedules can create additional stresses, challenges, and sacrifices for the caregiver and family and friends.

POTENTIAL HEALTH EFFECTS OF SHIFT WORK

The health effects of shift work are varied. Most caregivers who work rotating or unusual shifts adapt well over time, but may initially encounter physical, psychological, and social challenges associated with shift work. Caregivers who *choose* to work an unpopular shift for personal reasons tend to adapt better. Although shift work fits the lifestyle of many, the negative effects of shift work are well documented in the literature.

The Science Behind Sleep

The **circadian rhythm** is the body's 24-hour internal biological clock. It moderates physiological and psychological functions. In a normal work-during-day and sleep-during-night situation, people work when their circadian rhythm is high and sleep when it is low. People tend to be **larks** (i.e., morning people, who feel most alert and active during daylight hours) or **owls** (i.e., evening people, who feel most alert and active during the late afternoon and nighttime hours). Most individuals are neither extreme and are able to adapt to the necessary physical, psychosocial, and emotional changes related to working various shifts. Others may not cope well with shift work.

Sleep Deprivation

Nine hours of sleep is considered optimal for full daytime alertness. However, studies done on American day workers found that 7 to 8 hours is the average, with night-shift workers averaging 6.6 hours. **Sleep deprivation** (also called "sleep loss" or "sleep debt") is cumulative. The decreased alertness resulting from one night of insufficient sleep may not be noticeable, but the level of fatigue increases each night sleep deprivation occurs.

Sleep deprivation and extreme fatigue may be the greatest risk factor for injury related to shift work. When sleep-deprived, a caregiver may not be fully aware that work performance has deteriorated. Work tasks should be modified accordingly to maintain safety. Research suggests that the optimal mental performance level for workers occurs between 2 P.M. and 4 P.M. The lowest worker performance levels occur between 3:30 A.M. and 5:30 A.M.

Circadian rhythms affect work performance and alertness for those attempting to stay awake at night and interfere with sleep for those attempting to sleep during the day, contributing to sleep deprivation. Sleep deprivation may make it easier for caregivers to fall asleep at inappropriate times, thus affecting their ability to perform safely and efficiently. Two behaviors associated with fatigue—micro-sleep and automatic behavior syndrome—may occur both on and off the job, and both may increase injury risk. **Micro-sleep** is a brief nap that lasts from a few seconds to a few minutes. **Automatic behavior syndrome** is similar to micro-sleep, except that the eyes remain open and the person continues performing tasks.

IMPROVING CAREGIVER TOLERANCE FOR SHIFT WORK

Many health care facilities offer wellness programs to assist in coping with shift work and other challenges of caregiving. Some facilities also provide mental health resources such as Employee Assistance Programs (EAP) for times when additional help is needed.

Some employers have added wellness benefits to help offset the negative consequences that can accompany shift work. Examples of environmental changes that may improve performance for the shift worker include providing adequate fresh air and ventilation, bright light to increase alertness, variations in sound stimulus in contrast to routine monotonous sounds, pleasing aromas, and interesting tasks. Unfortunately, these strategies are not conducive to sleep for most clients, and therefore have limited practical application.

Many facilities have adopted forward shift rotation exclusively and are rotating less often. Studies suggest caregivers adjust more readily to **forward shift rotation,** in which rotating shift schedules advance in a clockwise direction (i.e., days to evenings, evenings to nights, nights to days, etc.). Research also suggests that cycling shift work no more often than every 21 days has been found to be most compatible with the caregiver's circadian rhythm.

Healthy Self-Care

Healthy self-care, including good sleep hygiene, maintaining regular physical activities, eating properly, and careful planning to accommodate the anticipated effects of shift work, can minimize negative consequences.

Sleep Hygiene

Sleep hygiene is essential to good health regardless of work schedule. For the caregiver working unusual shifts, examples of sleep hygiene activities may include:

- Going to sleep as soon as possible after a night shift.
- Adhering to a regular bedtime when working any shift.
- Avoiding depressants—e.g., sleep medications and alcohol.
- Avoiding stimulants—e.g., caffeine and nicotine.
- Making time for quiet relaxation before going to bed.
- Reminding family and friends of personal sleep and food needs due to shift work.
- Consuming the last caffeine at least 4 hours before you plan to sleep.
- Keeping the bedroom cool and dark for daytime sleeping.
- Creating a wake-up routine, just as there is for the average night sleeper.
- Using a fan to mask daytime noise.
- For the night-working caregiver, eating lightly throughout the shift with a moderate breakfast at the normal breakfast time to help avoid hunger during the day when sleep is needed.

Physical Activity

The caregiver should establish a regular physical exercise routine, optimally an hour of vigorous exercise throughout the day. Exercise should be avoided immediately before sleep. Physical exercise helps to maintain alertness. Physical fitness helps the caregiver cope with most challenges, not just challenges associated with shift work.

Nutrition and Fluid Intake

Drinking lots of water—not sodas and coffee—throughout the shift will help keep the body functioning at peak performance. In addition to increased fluids, consuming a variety of high-fiber foods, including raw vegetables and whole grains, helps to maintain good bowel function and will help the caregiver adapt to the digestive challenges that can accompany shift work. To further decrease gastrointestinal problems, eat slowly and chew food thoroughly. Cut back on foods highly seasoned with pepper, chili, curry, or mustard, and avoid fried foods and foods high in fat. For the evening-shift caregiver, eating the main meal in the middle of the day rather than the middle of the work shift may also help to minimize gastrointestinal problems that may be related to shift work.

THE AGING CAREGIVER AND SHIFT WORK

Tolerance to shift work declines with advancing age. Studies have found that persons older than 40 years have increased difficulties with shift work even when they had easily tolerated it in the past. Older workers may have more difficulty adjusting to working the night shift because of the circadian rhythm, and the older adult is more likely to be taking prescription drugs for medical conditions that may affect sleep. Effects of caffeine may linger up to 20 hours in the older worker, decreasing sleep quality and heightening morning drowsiness. If the older adult must work shifts, especially night shifts, the interventions mentioned previously in this chapter may lead to better adaptation.

CHAPTER

15

MANAGING STRESS IN THE CARE ENVIRONMENT

Defining Stress

Stress is tension linked to perceived pressure and anxiety, which cause a disturbance in a person's normal mental or physical state. **Eustress** is good stress; it helps a person perform better. **Distress** is stress that causes upset or makes a person sick. Both types of stress trigger the same automatic, immediate type of response.

Symptoms of Stress

Studies by NIOSH suggest that many symptoms may be early warning signs of workplace stress. (See Table 15-1.)

The Stress Response

The body has an automatic response when it perceives a **stressor**—a cause of stress. The stressor acts as a **trigger** to activate an automatic response that results in an outpouring of adrenaline, a stimulating hormone, into the bloodstream. This produces changes in the body that are intended to be protective, called "the fight-or-flight response."

TABLE 15-1   Early Warning Signs of Workplace Stress

Headaches	Sleep disturbances
Difficulty concentrating	Short temper
Upset stomach	Job dissatisfaction
Low morale	Muscle aches and pains
Drug and alcohol abuse	Depression
Domestic violence	Anxiety

Anxiety and the Fight-or-Flight Response

Anxiety is a response to perceived danger or threat. Scientifically, immediate or short-term anxiety is termed the **fight-or-flight response.** This reaction mobilizes the brain and sympathetic nervous system in response to a real (or perceived) threat. During the reaction, certain physical responses are generated. This reaction begins in the brain, when danger or fear is perceived, and sets off an automatic sequence of adaptive defense and escape responses. (See Table 15-2.)

General Adaptation Syndrome

In addition to the fight-or-flight response, other changes take place, called the **general adaptation syndrome (GAS).** GAS involves a secretion of **cortisol**

TABLE 15-2   Fight-or-Flight Response

Response	Purpose
Increasing heart rate and blood pressure	Increased blood to the muscles, brain, and heart
Faster breathing	Increased oxygen available for use
Tensing of muscles	Preparing muscles for action
Increasing mental alertness and sensitivity of sense organs (i.e., hearing, touch, smell)	Improves ability to assess the situation and act quickly
Increasing blood flow to the brain, heart, and muscles	Adequate blood supply and optimal central nervous system functioning are essential in preparing the body to respond. Added blood supply to muscles further prepares for physical response
Decreasing blood to digestive tract, kidneys, and liver	These organs are less important in times of crisis; blood supply is diverted from these organs to increase supply to heart, brain
Increasing blood sugar, fats, and cholesterol	Supplies extra energy
Rising platelets and blood clotting factors, decreasing blood flow to skin	Decreases bleeding in the event of an injury

by the adrenal glands. Cortisol has been called the "stress hormone," because blood cortisol levels are elevated during the normal response to stress.

The GAS consists of three stages: reaction to the alarm, resistance to the stressor, and exhaustion.

- Alarm—An alarm reaction occurs when the body is required to adapt to an external demand. The ability to resist a stressor is temporarily reduced, and is immediately followed by the fight-or–flight response.

- Resistance—The person tries using all internal resources to adapt. If the stress continues, the resources are exhausted and the ability to adapt decreases.

- Exhaustion—The person's internal resources are depleted. When the stress is over, the person may experience fatigue.

Each stage offers opportunities for intervention that can decrease the impact of the stressor on the individual. In situations of chronic, unremitting stress, physical and psychological problems can increase.

SOURCES OF STRESS

The conclusion drawn by many researchers studying the body's reaction to stress is that: *The way a person perceives a situation and how he or she handles that situation make all the difference in the amount of stress the person feels.* The immediate response people have to a situation is based on the way they are programmed to react. By understanding the power of perceptions, a person can learn to help break the cycle of stress.

There are four basic sources of stress:

1. Environment: Exposure to heat, cold, light, dark, traffic, and pollution.

2. Social stressors: Demands for time and attention, deadlines, financial problems, and loss of loved ones.

3. Physiological changes: Life transitions such as physiological changes of puberty, childbirth, changes resulting from a serious illness, surgery, or injury, and changes related to aging.

4. Thoughts: Attitudes and perceptions influence the way a person's brain interprets and translates events and determines when the fight-or-flight response will be activated. Instant reactions and self-talk such as "They shouldn't be doing that" or "I should be able to get this done" may trigger a stress response.

Potential Health Effects

The body remains on alert as long as the mind senses a threat. This accounts for some of the undesirable symptoms related to chronic stress:

- Rapid heartbeat
- Sweaty palms
- Tension headaches
- Digestive disorders
- Insomnia
- Weight gain or loss
- Weakened immune system

Short-lived or infrequent episodes of stress pose little health risk. However, when stress is unremitting, it can contribute to or aggravate long-term health problems.

Potential Adverse Effects of Excessive Stress on Health Care Workers

NIOSH defines *job stress* as "the harmful physical and emotional responses that occur when the requirements of the job do not match the capabilities, resources, or needs of the worker." Job stress can lead to poor health and even injury. Both NIOSH and the Centers for Disease Control and Prevention (CDC) report that occupational injuries can be related to stress. Stress-related occupational injuries may include:

- Musculoskeletal injuries related to muscle tension, such as a back injury resulting from overuse of tense muscles
- Walking into a cabinet or wall because attention was focused elsewhere
- Needle-stick injuries related to being distracted, anxious, or forgetful because of stress

Job Dissatisfaction and Stress

Job dissatisfaction is another aspect of job stress. If the caregiver is unable to manage his or her stress, it may lead to higher rates of emotional exhaustion and greater job dissatisfaction and burnout.

Stress and Burnout

When stress continues to escalate, job dissatisfaction, burnout, and health issues begin to appear. The term **burnout** is used to describe a state of fatigue and frustration among health care workers. Burnout is distinguished from general stress when the worker exhibits three behaviors related to work activities:

1. Emotional exhaustion—feeling drained and exhausted by work
2. Depersonalization—having negative or very detached feelings toward clients
3. Reduced personal accomplishments—work is suffering

Both individuals and work groups can show they are experiencing unmanageable levels of stress through a range of symptoms. Work group indicators of stress problems can include absenteeism, high or increased accident rates, poor or reduced work output, and poor interpersonal relations in the workplace.

Resiliency

Resilience is the ability to recover quickly from stressful situations. It is possible to become more resilient by developing a personal strategy to enhance resiliency and manage stress. Identifying and developing resources and strengths to effectively manage stressors have a positive effect on stress levels.

Building Resiliency

The following suggestions offered by the American Psychological Association may help caregivers adopt strategies to meet their personal needs:

1. Networking and good relationships with family members, friends, and coworkers are important. Accepting help and support helps strengthen resilience.
2. Avoid viewing a crisis as a hopeless problem. The crisis typically cannot be changed, but the caregiver may be able to change the way he or she interprets and responds to stressful events.
3. Accept change as part of living. Accept circumstances that cannot be changed and focus on circumstances that you can modify.
4. Develop realistic expectations.
5. Foster a positive view of yourself.
6. Keep things in perspective.

7. Develop a positive outlook.

8. Take care of yourself. Pay attention to your needs and feelings.

Managing Stress

Stress indicators include physical signs (dry mouth, fatigue), mental signs (forgetfulness, inability to concentrate), and psychological signs (anxiety, frustration, guilt, irritability, moodiness, nervousness, and tension).

Recognizing stress in others is often based on the *behavior* of the individual. Some of the common indicators of stress include substance abuse, emotional outbursts, excitability, restlessness, and trembling. Resistance to stress can be improved by improving physical fitness, practicing stress-reduction techniques, and improving time-management skills.

Physical Fitness

The caregiver should make a special effort to:

- Work in 60 minutes of vigorous exercise each day.

- Decrease or discontinue caffeine consumption.

- Eat well-balanced meals with fresh fruits, vegetables, and fiber. Lower your intake of foods high in sugars, fats, and carbohydrates.

- Get adequate restorative sleep.

Approaches to Stress Management

When the fight-or-flight mechanism takes over, the body is ready for action. In today's world, that physical action rarely accompanies stress. As a consequence, the individual's pulse rate stays up, he or she may be prone to rapid, shallow breathing, the heart beats faster, and muscles become tense with stored energy. The caregiver may try the following techniques in an effort to reduce these effects.

Time Management—Four Rules for Effective Time Management

Time-management strategies include:

- Set realistic expectations.

- Define priorities.

- Avoid distractions and lack of focus.

- Work at organizing personal and work life.

Imagery

Shut off the sounds and thoughts of the day to allow a 3-minute respite for the body and mind.

- Sit in a comfortable position, with your hands loosely touching in your lap. Lean back so that your back is supported by the chair.

- Close your eyes.

- Take a deep breath and slowly let it out.

- Remember a pleasant, quiet spot that you have enjoyed.

- Think about it in detail. What were the colors like? Could you feel a breeze on your face? Remember what it felt like to be relaxed and happy.

- Keep your breathing slow, deep, and controlled.

- After approximately 3 minutes, open your eyes and smile.

Relaxation Techniques

Exercises improve blood flow and can help reduce stress.

Deep Breathing

Deep breathing is an exercise that takes control of the breathing rate, gets additional oxygen into the body, and helps to slow the rapid heart rate.

- Sit in a comfortable position.

- Place a hand on your abdomen.

- Inhale slowly and deeply through your nose. Feel your abdomen rise. Hold your breath while you count to three.

- Exhale all your air slowly through your mouth while pursing your lips.

- Repeat the exercise at least two more times.

Stretching Exercises

Stretching exercises may help ease tension by increasing circulation.

Back Bend This exercise helps with relaxation and flexibility.

- Stand and clasp your hands behind your back. (Inhale)

- Slowly lean your upper body back without overarching your neck. Hold for 3 seconds. (Exhale)

- (Inhale) Slowly lean forward until you feel your low back muscles stretch. Hold for 3 seconds. (Exhale)
- Return to an upright, neutral position, and shake your hands at your side while you count to three.
- Repeat three times.

Neck Stretch

- Look straight ahead, arms at your side.
- Drop your left ear toward your left shoulder, don't raise the shoulder, and don't force your head over, let the weight of your head carry it as far as it wants to go.
- Take a deep breath.
- Hold for 3 seconds. Exhale slowly.
- Roll the head forward toward the right shoulder, and repeat the exercise on the right.
- Take a deep breath.
- Hold for 3 seconds. Exhale slowly and return to a neutral position, facing forward.
- Repeat the cycle three times.

Shoulder Stretch

- Extend your arms in front of you at shoulder height and interlace your fingers.
- Turn your palms outward. Lower your chin to your chest and extend your arms forward.
- Take a deep breath.
- Hold for 3 to 5 seconds. Exhale slowly.
- Return to a relaxed, neutral position, with your arms at your side. Wiggle your fingers while you count to three.
- Repeat three times.

HUMOR

Humor is a stress reducer; there are many additional ways to relieve stress. Any activity that creates a change of scene, uses up some energy, and is enjoyable will do. Take a walk, ride a bike, have a picnic lunch. Spend time with your family and friends. Get a massage, go to a movie. Help a friend.

Play with your dog. Fly a kite. The possibilities are endless. The goal is the same: When you are feeling stressed, find an activity that allows your body to recover from the side effects of stress.

SOURCES OF HELP

It is important for caregivers experiencing workplace stress beyond their control to discuss the issues with the supervisor. It is unrealistic to assume that any workplace will be totally free of stress, but every employer has a responsibility to reduce the level of stress in the workplace so that it is manageable.

Employee Assistance Programs

Employee Assistance Programs (EAPs) are employer-sponsored programs set up to help the caregiver handle personal and emotional problems that are interfering with work performance.

Stress-Management Programs

Training programs can include coping techniques such as muscle relaxation, meditation, and time management. Employers may also introduce lifestyle training into the workplace through pamphlets or newsletters that give information about health, exercise, and diet.

Support Groups

The EAP may recommend support groups of benefit to the caregiver. Such groups may be sponsored by nonprofit organizations, faith-based organizations, or local agencies. Support groups such as 12-Step recovery programs (Alcoholics Anonymous, Al-Anon, Codependents Anonymous) may offer a source of help to the caregiver, especially if substance abuse is a problem. However, participation in these groups should not be limited to those caregivers struggling with substance abuse. Caregivers may benefit from these groups as a forum for improving coping capacity by improving communication and conflict-resolution skills.

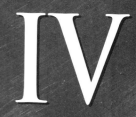

SECTION IV

IMPROVING WORKING CONDITIONS IN HEALTH CARE

C H A P T E R

16

INFLUENCING CHANGE

SAFETY CULTURE

A **safety culture** can be described as the values, attitudes, competencies, and behaviors of individuals and groups that establish the commitment, structure, and depth of a safety program within an organization. Characteristics of a positive safety culture include communication founded on mutual trust, shared ideas of the importance of safety, and confidence in sound preventive measures.

FACTORS LEADING TO A POSITIVE SAFETY CULTURE

A positive safety culture is one in which individuals at all levels of an organization work together to create a work environment where caregivers are confident of their own safety and that of their clients. Studies suggest that certain factors create the foundation of a positive safety culture. These factors include:

- The commitment at all levels of leadership, including the chief executive

- The involvement of employees

- Knowledge of gaps in competent practice

- Effective communications

- Commonly understood and agreed-upon goals
- Feedback after implementation of new ideas
- Seeking knowledge from lessons learned
- Continual attention to workplace safety and health
- Encouragement of a questioning attitude by all individuals

Model for Influencing Change

The **Influencing Change Model** (see Figure 16-1) focuses on a continuum of three components that can best lead to change, including assessment, intervention, and feedback. The model is intended to provide a framework to help groups identify, diagnose, and resolve problems as they occur.

Group process consultation is the reasoned and intentional intervention by a consultant or facilitator into ongoing events and dynamics of a group with the purpose of helping that group effectively attain its agreed-upon objectives.

In the assessment phase, the group process consultant works with a caregiver group to gather information related to such things as the current culture, behaviors, needed skills, background of the practice in need of changing, and any barriers that stand in the way of the need to change.

Depending upon the assessment outcome, the consultant may suggest one or a variety of interventions. Reddy suggests that idea generation, skills training, reflection, and interpretive discussions are among the different types of interventions that might be successful.

The consultant provides feedback to the group of caregivers as they work through the various interventions and begin to move toward the needed changes. The feedback should be given at the earliest opportunity,

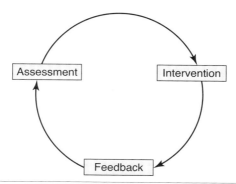

FIGURE 16-1 Influencing Change Model. *(Adapted from Intervention Skills by W. Brendan Reddy, 1994)*

and should focus on behaviors that can be changed. The group receiving the information should be willing to listen, to respond nondefensively, to check out the data with others, and to consider changing the behavior.

This Influencing Change Model is effective in creating a positive environment for cultural change by encouraging each participant to share input.

Communication Strategies to Prevent Injuries

Communication among caregivers is critical to creating and maintaining a positive safety culture. Some health care organizations provide training focused on how caregivers can "watch out" for one another and their clients, including information on how to speak up when observing high-risk behavior. Such open and collaborative communication helps prevent mishaps and injuries. Other key points in effective communication include the following:

- Recognize one's own obstacles to communication.

- Share information.

- Encourage open communication between caregivers.

- Stop what you are doing and give the person your undivided attention.

When a caregiver encounters a hazard, that person must take responsibility to communicate with the supervisor or other persons who can fix the problem if the caregiver cannot do it alone.

Feedback as a Method of Preventing Injuries

Communication processes are completed when active listening has taken place and feedback has been received. Feedback can come in the form of praise (i.e., reinforcement) for behaviors that are appreciated and valued or **constructive feedback** (i.e., coaching) for undesirable behaviors for which change is sought. In a positive safety culture, praise and constructive feedback occur freely among peers as well as between supervisors and caregivers.

Praise can occur in public. By providing praise in public, the good behaviors and skills being recognized are observed and validated by others, increasing the likelihood that the positive behavior will be repeated. However, constructive feedback for behaviors that should be changed is best done in private as soon as possible after witnessing the behavior. This process of providing feedback links the discussion with the behavior, reducing the risk of the individual taking the comments personally and becoming defensive. Feedback is needed when performing any new procedure, such as learning to use a new piece of equipment for safe client movement.

Injury Prevention through Supervision Supervision is used to monitor desired behaviors as well as to develop measures to assess effectiveness of safety interventions. Communicating job expectations and physical requirements to the caregiver is an important part of supervision. The supervisor conducts reviews to evaluate the way a task is performed, including the appropriateness of the equipment used.

Orientation and continuing education for caregivers, supervisors, and other leaders is required to keep everyone up to date on safety requirements and expectations. Working together, supervisors and caregivers can build a positive safety culture and help to prevent injuries.

Injury Prevention through Training Effective training is an important administrative control to prevent injuries. It is necessary for all caregivers to receive training on any new or redesigned physical work tasks in order to prevent injuries and maintain quality care. Training is most effective when it includes a combination of classroom education and supervised hands-on practice.

A health care system with a positive safety culture involves caregivers and others in promptly identifying and controlling hazards, facilitating change and communication, and providing feedback. Influencing and changing culture takes time and energy, but the benefits can be rewarding for all involved.

CHAPTER

17

GETTING INVOLVED

THE IMPORTANCE OF PUBLIC EDUCATION

In 2002, the Joint Commission appointed a group of physicians, nurses, pharmacists, and other client safety experts to identify client safety concerns. These recommendations became known as the Joint Commission **National Patient Safety Goals (NPSGs),** and compliance with these goals became a requirement for Joint Commission accreditation. (See Table 17-1.) This requirement and increased media attention related to medical errors have created public awareness related to client safety concerns in health care facilities. A similar phenomenon is needed regarding the interrelatedness of caregiver safety and client safety. As public attention is drawn to the importance of a safe work environment in health care, safety education occurs. As safety education improves, the public becomes better able to identify hazards and unsafe work practices, and more likely to partner with health care organizations to implement evidence-based controls.

EMPLOYEE RIGHTS AND RESPONSIBILITIES UNDER OSHA

As discussed in earlier chapters, the Occupational Safety and Health Act of 1970 mandates that employers identify and eliminate or control workplace hazards. The Occupational Health and Safety Administration (OSHA) standards prescribe specific workplace controls the employer must adopt. However, this

TABLE 17-1 Examples of 2007 Joint Commission National Patient Safety Goals

Improve the accuracy of patient identification.

Improve the effectiveness of communication among caregivers.

Reduce the risk of health care–associated infections.

Reduce the risk of patient harm resulting from falls.

Reduce the risk of surgical fires.

Source: Joint Commission National Patient Safety Goals, http://www.jointcommission.org/PatientSafety/NationalPatientSafetyGoals/.

Act also specifically directs employees to comply with all OSHA standards. Employees are given certain rights and responsibilities under OSHA, as well. Employee rights under OSHA are summarized in Table 17-2. Employees are encouraged to be active in the employers' safety and health

TABLE 17-2 Employee Rights under OSHA

Employees have the right to:

- Review copies of OSHA-provided standards, rules, and regulations,
- Request information from the employer on safety and health hazards in the workplace, precautions to take, and procedures to follow if involved in an accident or exposure to toxic substances,
- Access to relevant employee exposure and medical records,
- Request an OSHA inspection if you believe hazardous conditions or violations of standards exist,
- Accompany an OSHA compliance officer during the inspection tour, or have an authorized employee representative do so,
- Respond to questions from the OSHA compliance officer,
- Observe monitoring or measuring of hazardous materials and see the resulting records,
- Review or have an authorized representative review the employer's Log of Work-Related Occupational Injuries and Illnesses (OSHA 300) at a reasonable time and in a reasonable manner,
- Object to the time frame set by OSHA for the employer to correct a violation by writing to the OSHA area director within 15 working days from the date the employer receives the citation,
- Submit a written request to the National Institute for Occupational Safety and Health (NIOSH) about whether any substance in the workplace has potentially toxic effects in the concentration being used, and, if requested, have your name withheld from the employer,
- Be notified if the employer applies for a variance from an OSHA standard, and have an opportunity to testify at a variance hearing and appeal the final decision,
- Have your name withheld from the employer, by request to OSHA, if you sign and file a written complaint,
- Be advised of OSHA actions regarding a complaint, and request an informal review of any decision not to inspect the site or issue a citation,
- File a complaint if punished or discriminated against for acting as a "whistle-blower" under the OSH Act or 13 other federal statutes for which OSHA has jurisdiction or for refusing to work when faced with imminent danger of death or serious injury and there is insufficient time for OSHA to inspect.

Source: Occupational Safety and Health Act of 1970, Pub. L. 91-596, §2193.

TABLE 17-3   Employee Responsibilities under OSHA

- Read the OSHA poster at the job site.
- Comply with all applicable OSHA standards.
- Follow all lawful employer safety and health rules and regulations, and wear or use prescribed protective equipment while working.
- Report hazardous conditions to the supervisor.
- Report any job-related injury or illness to the employer, and seek treatment promptly.
- Cooperate with the OSHA compliance officer conducting an inspection if he or she inquires about safety and health conditions in the workplace.
- Exercise rights under the OSH Act in a responsible manner.

Source: Occupational Safety and Health Act of 1970, Pub. L. 91-596, §2193.

activities. Developing open communication and relationships based on mutual respect will be of benefit when safety and health concerns arise. Most employers are willing to listen and adapt working environments to address safety concerns.

Employee responsibilities are summarized in Table 17-3. Caregivers may be unaware of their regulatory responsibilities regarding safe working conditions. Employee education should include information regarding these rights and responsibilities and how the caregiver can get involved in the organizational safety effort.

CAREGIVER INVOLVEMENT IN THE SAFETY EFFORT

Although the employer has the legal obligation to inform the caregiver of health hazards in the workplace and to implement the appropriate controls, a safe working environment cannot be created without the caregiver's participation in using safe work practices and making the most effective use of the controls. The caregiver—not the employer—is most likely to observe an unsafe working condition or a potential hazard. Many hazards cannot be corrected unless they are reported. The caregiver plays an important part in helping to create a safe environment. Caregiver involvement is absolutely essential.

Labor Organizations and Safety

Labor organizations are in a unique position to advocate for safe working conditions. Union members working with management in a cooperative manner can bring about rapid safety improvements. In fact, the Occupational Safety and Health Act of 1970 was the result, in part, of labor organization efforts to improve workplace safety and overall working conditions. Labor organizations such as the American Nurses Association and Service Employees International Union are often involved in lobbying efforts to improve working conditions through legislative action.

Professional Associations

Professional associations are an excellent source of safety information and advocacy. Most association Web sites have a link to specific safety and health information for their members and many have strong governmental affairs committees that work to keep members informed and to lobby for change.

Safety Committee

Regulatory requirements for employee safety committees differ slightly from state to state but have the same intent. In many states, OSHA requires that most employers under OSHA jurisdiction create a formal safety committee; staff-level participation is expected. The Joint Commission does not require organizations to have a safety committee, but it does require that multi-disciplinary improvement teams meet to address safety concerns. These Joint Commission committees are often called "Environment of Care Committees."

The OSHA safety committee is typically composed of employer representatives, employee representatives, and, if applicable, labor organization representatives. A safety committee is often considered a trademark of an effective safety program, but the committee does not make the program effective. Effective safety programs are the result of employee and management commitment and involvement at all levels, not just within the safety committee.

CHAPTER

18

STAYING INFORMED: FINDING RELIABLE INFORMATION

Staying informed is a professional and personal responsibility for caregivers and is essential to maintaining client and caregiver safety and health. This chapter provides an overview of the regulatory and nonregulatory federal agencies, professional associations, and colleges and universities that serve as major resources for this type of information. Web-site addresses are provided. (Consult the text on which this guide is based, *Working Safely in Health Care: A Practical Guide,* for additional information on accessing these Web sites.)

REGULATORY AGENCIES

A **regulatory agency** is a government agency dedicated to an area of specialized expertise and an assignment to develop and enforce laws, rules, standards, regulations, or other orders authorized by the legislative process. The rules established by regulatory agencies are mandatory. It is common for state and local regulatory agencies to have more stringent rules. Generally the more stringent rule is the one that must be followed.

Examples of regulatory agencies that help to protect caregivers are provided. These agencies have Web sites and toll-free numbers that caregivers can use to get information about current and developing regulations.

Occupational Safety and Health Administration

The Occupational Safety and Health Administration (OSHA) (www.osha.gov) has been mentioned extensively in earlier chapters. Although the Bloodborne Pathogens standard is the one most familiar to caregivers, there are many other OSHA standards that apply to health care settings.

OSHA maintains an extensive Web site to assist the public. The OSHA Web site also includes "e-Tools," which are Web-based training features related to specific hazards or industries. These "e-Tools" are interactive, and provide interesting information that can be used for training about hazard identification and control. (See Figure 18-1.)

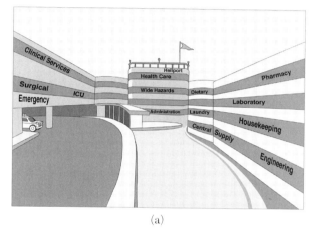

(a)

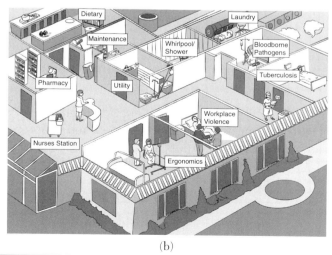

(b)

FIGURE 18-1 *Hospital and nursing home e-Tools are interactive Web-based training tools designed by the Occupational Health and Safety Administration to help the caregiver find reliable health and safety information. (a) Hospital e-Tool; (b) Nursing Home e-Tool.*

Employment Standards Administration

The Employment Standards Administration (ESA) (http://www.dol.gov) is the Department of Labor agency with the mission to enhance the welfare and protect the rights of American workers, particularly as they relate to hours and conditions of work.

Equal Employment Opportunity Commission

The Equal Employment Opportunity Commission (EEOC) (http://www.eeoc.gov) provides information to caregivers and other employees who believe they are subject to discrimination by their employer.

OTHER FEDERAL RESOURCES

Federal agencies and organizations develop guidelines that health care facilities may adopt and integrate into care delivery. State governments may have the authority to make adherence to these guidelines mandatory, so although a *federal* agency may not be authorized to require that a guideline be followed, a counterpart *state* or *local* agency may make a certain federal guideline mandatory in its jurisdiction. Examples of these agencies are provided.

U.S. Public Health Service

The U.S. Public Health Service (USPHS) (http://www.usphs.gov/) operates within the Department of Health and Human Services (DHHS). The USPHS mission is to provide highly trained and mobile health care professionals to carry out programs to promote the health of the nation, understand and prevent disease and injury, and furnish health expertise in time of war or other national or international emergencies.

Two divisions of the USPHS that have significant impact on health care workers are the Centers for Disease Control and Prevention (CDC) and the National Institute for Occupational Safety and Health (NIOSH).

Centers for Disease Control and Prevention

CDC (http://www.cdc.gov) is recognized worldwide as an authority on communicable diseases and provides recommendations for caregivers about immunizations, precautions to prevent transmission of infectious diseases, hand-washing protocols, and other topics intended to reduce risk in health care facilities.

National Institute for Occupational Safety and Health

NIOSH (http://www.cdc.gov/niosh) is the federal agency responsible for conducting research and making recommendations for the prevention of work-related injury and illness. NIOSH is part of the CDC.

Agency for Healthcare Research and Quality

The Agency for Healthcare Research and Quality (AHRQ) (http://www.ahrq .gov) supports health services research that will improve the quality of health care and promote evidence-based decision making at the bedside. The AHRQ publishes this research in the form of articles and guidelines that can be quickly transferred to practice.

Department of Homeland Security

The Department of Homeland Security (DHS) (http://www.dhs.gov) can provide multiple resources to draw upon as caregivers consider their role in responding to mass casualty events, terrorist attacks, or other events that threaten national security. The DHS frequently refers users to CDC, the Environmental Protection Agency, and other government agency Web sites in these events and may be a gateway to other information when disaster strikes.

Bureau of Labor Statistics

The Bureau of Labor Statistics (BLS) (http://www.bls.gov) is the principal fact-finding agency for the federal government in the broad field of labor economics and statistics.

Workers' Compensation Information

The North Carolina Industrial Commission provides a complete list of U.S. workers' compensation agencies in each state on its Web site (http://www .comp.state.nc.us/).

PROFESSIONAL ORGANIZATIONS

Professional organizations offer caregivers opportunities to learn about occupational safety and health from various perspectives.

American Association of Occupational Health Nurses

The American Association of Occupational Health Nurses (AAOHN) (http://www.aaohn.org/) consists of nurses whose practice area is safety and health within the worker population for a variety of settings, including industry, manufacturing, office settings, and health care facilities.

American College of Occupational and Environmental Medicine

The American College of Occupational and Environmental Medicine (ACOEM) (http://www.acoem.org/) is an international specialty organization whose practice specialty is the prevention and management of injury, illness, and disability related to occupational and environmental factors.

American Industrial Hygiene Association

Founded in 1939, the American Industrial Hygiene Association (AIHA) (http://www.aiha.org) is a particularly good resource for those seeking information about specific chemicals in health care work sites.

American Nurses Association

The American Nurses Association (ANA) (http://www.nursingworld.org/) participates in policy initiatives to change and improve health care quality and working conditions and provides professional continuing education opportunities for members.

American Public Health Association (APHA)

The American Public Health Association (APHA) (http://www.apha.org/) focuses on a broad set of issues affecting individual and environmental health, including communicable disease control, smoking cessation, maternal–child health, ergonomics, and other occupational health issues.

American Society of Safety Engineers

The American Society of Safety Engineers (ASSE) (http://www.asse.org/) can be called upon to recognize safety hazards, identify control measures, and measure outcomes of hazard-abatement efforts.

Association of Occupational Health Professionals in Healthcare

The Association of Occupational Health Professionals in Healthcare (AOHP) (http://www.aohp.org/about/home.asp) is a national organization for occupational health professionals from many disciplines who practice in health care settings. It is primarily an educational and professional development organization for its members.

Association for Practitioners in Infection Control and Epidemiology

The Association for Practitioners in Infection Control and Epidemiology (APIC) (http://www.apic.org/) focuses primarily on health care–associated infections and infection-control efforts to protect clients; in recent years they have also taken positions regarding the protection of health care workers exposed to certain communicable diseases.

Center for American Nurses

The Center for American Nurses (CAN) (http://centerforamericannurses .org/) serves individual, nonunion nurses by providing programs, tools, services, and strategies designed to make nurses their own best advocates in their practice environments.

Joint Commission

The Joint Commission (http://www.jointcommission.org/) has pledged to provide caregivers and others with information, guidance, and access to training resources focused on protecting employees' health and safety. Most of the employee-focused materials are listed under the performance improvement area of the Web site.

UNIONS AND LABOR ORGANIZATIONS

A number of unions offer information to caregivers. Examples of unions that represent caregivers are noted here; many others are also interested in providing information to caregivers and enhancing safety and health among health care workers.

American Federation of State, County, and Municipal Employees

American Federation of State, County, and Municipal Employees (AFSCME) (http://www.afscme.org/) focuses its efforts on health care–related hazards such as workplace violence, infectious diseases, ergonomic hazards, and others.

Service Employees International Union

The Service Employees International Union (SEIU) (http://www.seiu.org/) produces resources such as posters, films, books, and brochures on current topics that affect caregivers.

United American Nurses, American Federation of Labor and Congress of Industrial Organizations

The United American Nurses (UAN), American Federation of Labor and Congress of Industrial Organizations (AFL-CIO) (http://www.uan.org/) is the largest union for registered nurses in the United States. Resources for caregivers include leadership training and information about working conditions, staffing, wages, and ergonomics issues.

COLLEGES AND UNIVERSITIES

NIOSH is associated with several universities throughout the United States, designated as Education and Research Centers (ERCs). The ERCs that offer continuing educational courses that are listed on the NIOSH Web site.

The University of Virginia has established the International Healthcare Worker Safety Center, which hosts EPINet (http://www.healthsystem .virginia.edu/internet/epinet/). The EPINet details which categories of workers are getting injured, how the injuries occur, where on the body most needlesticks occur, and other useful data that can be used to assess the risk to caregivers. This site also provides links to the newest innovations in safer devices.

The Oregon Health and Science University Center for Research on Occupational and Environmental Toxicology (CROET) (http://www .croetweb.com/) provides information on a number of hazards that caregivers may encounter, including back injuries and emergency response issues, and there is a specific page for "Healthcare" on its Web site.

CHAPTER

19

SHOPPING FOR A SAFE EMPLOYER

FINDING THE RIGHT
HEALTH CARE ENVIRONMENT

Although it seems like a simple process, selecting a health care career environment may not be as easy as it looks.

Deciding Where to Start

When evaluating the health care setting for employment consideration, it is important to consider the type of schedules that are typically offered to caregivers in each setting, the primary job tasks assigned to caregivers by the prospective employer, and the interaction that is expected between the caregiver and the client. It is helpful to create a file or a notebook to keep track of potential employers or health care settings that are appealing.

Research and Documentation

There are a number of places where a potential employee can search for key information about a prospective employer, and this step should not be skipped. The information gathered can help the caregiver determine whether the facility is a safe place to work, but also may provide clues as to the quality of care provided in the facility.

Occupational Safety and Health Administration Compliance Inspection History

The Occupational Safety and Health Administration (OSHA) has a link within its Web site that allows anyone to inquire as to whether an employer has had an OSHA compliance inspection. This online system provides information on violations and penalties connected with listed inspections. The caregiver can search the system by establishment.

Joint Commission

The Joint Commission conducts accreditation surveys that may provide clues to organizational culture. The Joint Commission has a program called "Quality Check" that provides accreditation and comparison information that people can use to determine whether a health care organization will meet their needs.

Magnet Hospital Designation

The American Nurse Credentialing Center (ANCC) provides oversight for the Magnet Hospital program. Magnet status is considered to be a benchmark for quality nursing care. The ANCC Web site allows access to the listing of Magnet-credentialed facilities.

State Agencies

State agencies often handle the state accreditation process (often referred to as the "state survey process") for long-term care facilities. The specific agency involved varies from state to state, but is most often a function of the Department of Health and Human Services within the state. Contact the state's agency directory to connect with the appropriate agency. If survey information is available, it should be used in evaluating potential employers.

Personal Inquiries

Make a list of people whom you could contact as part of your research process. It is best if you know these individuals personally and can contact them without breaching confidentiality rules or personal privacy. This list may include friends, family, or peers who are familiar with the employer, current or past clients you know personally, and employees.

It is important to develop a list of questions that will provide key information for the selection of potential employers. Questions for a client or a client's family might include:

- Do you enjoy the facility?

- Are the employees friendly and helpful?

- Have you developed friendships with the employees who care for you?

- Do the employees change frequently?
- Are your needs and concerns addressed quickly?
- If you had the chance, would you stay at this facility or move to another facility?

Questions for an employee you know personally might include:

- Do you like working at this facility?
- Does the management value and support safety for both the employees and the clients?
- Is your opinion valued?
- Does the environment support open, candid discussion of important issues related to client care and caregiver working conditions?
- Do employees stay at this facility for a while, or is there a lot of turnover?
- Do you receive the training you feel is necessary to do your job effectively and safely?
- Is the equipment available that you feel is necessary to do your job effectively and safely?

Public Records, Publications, and News Articles

A background search on potential employers would not be complete without looking into public records, publications, and news articles. Selecting information from widely known, reputable reporting agencies such as those discussed in earlier chapters will provide key facts that can later be used in developing questions to ask a potential employer if the opportunity to interview for a position arises.

THE INTERVIEW

An interview presents another opportunity to learn more about the employer. After the applicant answers the questions that have been asked by the prospective employer, there is often an opportunity for the applicant to ask any lingering questions. This is the time to learn more about the employer, and discover how important workplace safety is in their facility.

Key Characteristics

Organizations that put a priority on safety are proud of their efforts and share this type of information with the community, clients, employees, and prospective employees. They may offer an opportunity to view their **Log of Work-Related Injuries and Illnesses (OSHA 300 log)** and **sharps**

injury log, both of which are required for most health care facilities covered by OSHA.

The OSHA 300 log is used to classify work-related injuries and illnesses and to note the extent and severity of each case. When an incident occurs that meets certain criteria, most employers covered by OSHA are required to use the log to record specific details about what happened and how it happened. The Summary is a separate form (Form 300A) that shows the totals for the year in each of six categories:

- Injuries

- Skin disorders

- Respiratory conditions

- Poisonings

- Hearing loss

- All other illnesses

At the end of the year, the employer is required to post the Summary in a visible location so that employees are aware of the injuries and illnesses occurring in their workplace. Employees have the right to review these injury and illness records. Time loss or modified work is also captured on the Summary, and may provide clues related to injury severity.

The sharps injury log is used for recording percutaneous injuries from contaminated sharps. The information in the sharps injury log must be recorded by the employer and maintained in such a manner as to protect the confidentiality of the injured employee. The sharps injury log shall contain, at a minimum:

- The type and brand of device involved in the incident

- The department or work area where the exposure incident occurred

- An explanation of how the incident occurred

A safe employer may also be willing to discuss its program for bringing injured workers back to work. These employers often make an effort to bring the employee back as soon as the attending physician has determined it safe to do so, even if duties must be modified to prevent aggravating the injured part as healing continues. Prompt return to work hastens recovery and allows the caregiver to remain productive until the physician has provided a work release allowing a return to unrestricted duties.

Key Observations

Arriving early for an interview gives the hiring and Human Resources staff an early indication of the candidate's interest in the position and provides candidates a good amount of time to observe the activities in the facility.

Interaction between facility staff and clients is a key observation. Do staff members appear happy and calm, or hurried and stressed? Do they communicate in a method that is respectful of others? An interview candidate may observe some or all of the following while in the facility:

Are aisles and hallways free of tripping hazards?

Are floor surfaces (tile, carpet, etc.) well maintained and in good condition?

If the entry to the building has a solid surface floor, are there any spills or wet spots?

Are employees carrying large, heavy, or awkward loads?

If clients can be observed, are they assisted in any way by the employees?

Do employees assist clients manually (by physically lifting or transferring) or with equipment and appropriate safe client handling devices?

Is the building in fair to good condition, or does it appear to be rundown and poorly maintained?

Are employees talking about other employees? Is the tone of the conversation respectful?

Ultimately, candidates will likely be able to determine from their observations and the interview whether they can envision themselves working happily and successfully in the environment. If the answer is "no," this should weigh heavily in the decision to accept a job if an offer is extended.

Key Questions

It is important to go into the interview with a short list of key questions to ask after the employer has finished asking questions.

Questions for the potential employer might include:

1. *Do you have a safety committee? If so, what is the role of your safety committee?* Safety committees may be required by OSHA in some states, or by collective bargaining agreements. The function of a safety committee is to create and maintain interest in injury prevention and to help initiate and maintain communication between management, nonsupervisory employees, and organized labor, if applicable.

2. *How are client needs and medical conditions recorded and communicated to the appropriate staff and caregivers?* Letting the potential employer describe the process will provide good insight into their communication and documentation procedures.

3. *What equipment is available to assist the clients who are partially weight-bearing or dependent? What percentage of the clients in this facility are totally dependent? Partially dependent? Independent? What is the policy for assisting clients from the floor?* Learning about the facility's safe client handling and movement program and the equipment used for moving clients will provide insight into their willingness to invest in new technology and methods.

4. *What safety training is provided to employees?* Thorough training should be provided at the time of hire and periodically thereafter. Ask how this training is accomplished and how often.

5. *How do you encourage employees to work safely, and how are they involved in the safety process?* Ask if caregivers are invited to work on safety improvement teams. Ask about safety suggestion programs. Ask about systems in place to reward employees for safe behaviors and helping to identify and correct hazards. Employee involvement may include a safety suggestion box, a safety observation process, or a safety article or newsletter.

SAFETY ON THE JOB

The first 6 months on the job are the most critical for the success and safety of the new employee. Caregivers should ask their managers to describe the training that will be provided. This is a perfect time to ask questions about safety training and make sure there is a clear understanding of the on-the-job performance expectations. To help ensure that an on-the-job injury or incident does not occur, ask who should be contacted if there are questions regarding employee and client safety or if a hazard is observed. When in doubt about a procedure or policy, always ask before acting.

Getting Involved in Safety

As a new employee, getting involved in the safety committee might be more difficult because of the need to focus work hours on learning the various aspects and tasks of the job. Express an interest in joining a safety committee or other workplace safety group, and at a minimum ask to be provided copies of information that those committees or groups generate.

On-the-Job Injuries

As mentioned earlier, most facilities with a successful safety system will have a program to bring injured workers back to modified or transitional work during the healing process whenever feasible. The job modification must be approved by the medical provider treating the injury. This **transitional work** is generally defined as a temporary modified work assignment within the employee's physical abilities, knowledge, and skills. Transitional positions minimize time away from work, which typically lessens the financial burden for the caregiver and the employer, and promotes rehabilitation. Ultimately, the sooner caregivers return to work, the sooner they will heal and continue to progress in their careers.

INDEX

N

Near-miss incidents, 8
Needlestick Safety and Prevention
    Act, 129
Negative pressure room, 115
Nephrotoxins, 85
Neurotoxins, 85
Neutral postures, 24–27
N-95 respirators, 115, 120
Nuclear weapons, 155
Nutrition, 162, 169

O

Obesity, 57
Occupational Safety and Health Administration
    (OSHA), 4–6, 109, 191
    HazCom, 85
    rights, 186–188
    training, 132
On-call workers, 166
Outpatients
    airborne precautions, 116
    droplet precautions, 116–117
Outsole, 80
Owls, 167

P

Pathogens, 106, 128–132
Patient Safety Center, 59–74
Percutaneous exposure, 107
Permissible exposure limit (PEL), 90
Personal protective equipment (PPE), 11–12,
    24, 110, 119–122
Physical hazards, 12
Pointing devices, 34–35
Pollutant emissions, 97
Portable floor-based lifts, 54
Portable lifts, 47–48
Portal of entry, 105, 107
Portal of exit, 105, 106
Postexposure prophylaxis (PEP), 123
Postincident violence, 145–146
Powered transport devices, 48
Preassault phase, 141
Preparedness, 148–149
Prevention
    fire, 157–158
    hazards, 3
    injuries, 184
    WRMSDs, 23–24
Preventive maintenance, 101
Preventive medical care, 165
Professional associations, 189
Professional organizations, 193–195
Protective clothing, 119
Psychological factors, 76
Psychosocial hazards, 13
Public education, 186
Pulling, 29

Pushing, 29
Pyrophorics, 85

R

Radiological materials, 153–154
Reactivity data, 91
Recovery, 149
Recreational health hazards, 161
Re-entrainment, 100
Reflective communication, 142
Regulations
    disease transmission, 109
    regulatory agencies, 190–192
Relaxation techniques, 177–178
Repetition, reducing, 31–32
Reporting
    pathogens, 132–133
    exposure, 108
Reservoir, 105, 106
Resiliency, 175–176
Respirators, 115, 120–122
Respiratory protection, 120–122
Response
    emergency management, 149, 155–157
    fight-or-flight, 172
    of stress, 171–172
Risk
    assessing, 8–12
    of client injury, 46–52
    client movement, 51–52
    falls, reducing, 76–80
    of hazards, 7–8
    pathogens, 129
    violence, 138–140
    WRMSDs, 19–23
Room cleaning, 41
Rotating shifts, 166
Routes of exposure, 87, 91–92

S

Safe client movement, 45–46
    airborne precautions, 116
    algorithms, 60–74
    assessment, 59–60
    bariatric care, 57–59
    droplets, 116–117
    functional ability, 51–52
    hierarchy of controls, 52–57
    Patient Safety Center, 59–74
    risk of injury, 46–52
Safe handling, 92
Safe sharps, selection of, 131
Safety, 202–203
    caregivers, 188–189
    chemical. See Chemical safety
    committees, 189
    disease transmission, 123–126
    emergency management, 155–157
    job safety analysis (JSA), 9